holistic assessment
of the
healthy aged

holistic assessment of the healthy aged

Miriam Martin Schrock, R.N., M.S.
Assistant Professor
College of Nursing
The University of Iowa
Iowa City, Iowa

A WILEY MEDICAL PUBLICATION
JOHN WILEY & SONS
New York • Chichester • Brisbane • Toronto

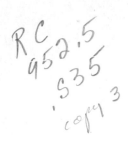
Credits

Chapter 1, page 1; Chapter 4, page 88
© The Washington Post, March 16, 1975. Reprinted with permission.

Chapter 3, page 51
From THE NEW INTERNATIONAL VERSION, Copyright © 1978 by: The New York
International Bible Society. Used by permission of Zondervan Publishing House.

Library of Congress Cataloging in Publication Data:

Schrock, Miriam Martin.

Holistic assessment of the healthy aged.

(A Wiley medical publication)
Includes index.
1. Geriatrics. 2. Aged. 3. Holistic medicine.
4. Gerontology. I. Title.
RC952.5.S35   618.97   80-10198
ISBN 0-471-05597-2

Printed in the United States of America

10 9 8 7 6 5 4 3 2 1

*To my Grandmother Eberly, who demonstrated the goodness
of aging by the way she lived*

contributors

Marie Cassamassimo Faynor, R.N., M.S.
Formerly Assistant Professor
College of Nursing
The University of Iowa

W. Stanley Good, M.S.S.W.
Associate Professor
School of Social Work
The University of Iowa

Toni Tripp-Reimer, R.N., Ph.D.
Assistant Professor
College of Nursing
The University of Iowa

foreword

The focus of health care is on illness or so says the American health care scene. Prepaid health insurance programs reward sickness, not wellness and the behaviors that promote it. However, today's baccalaureate-prepared nurse is as concerned with wellness as he or she is with illness.

What is wellness care? Few resources are yet available to define this new role for nurses. The teacher who sets out to make this the focus of the curriculum finds few aids available. This book helps fill that void by discussing wellness care for a specific age group in our population.

Wellness care is relevant to people of all ages. Contrary to the thinking of many, it is highly relevant to the aged population. Many people see old age as a time when chronic illness ends a previous state of wellness. This book rightly sets forth the fact that the vast majority of older people enjoy a relatively well state of health. Moreover, as the aged constantly increase in numbers in our society, concern for their health becomes an increasingly greater area of focus of nursing and nursing curricula. This book is welcome not only for its exploration of wellness care but also for its application to an age group with whom nursing students in a baccalaureate program frequently begin their clinical experience.

The second emphasis of the book is on viewing older people holistically. For some time in the nursing profession we have realized that people are more than biological beings whose physical bodies need sustenance and repair. Psychosocial needs have received a great deal of attention in nursing curricula. Recently nursing professionals have become more aware that people are cultural and spiritual beings, and that these dimensions must be understood also if people are to have their individual needs met in ways that are acceptable to them.

Holism involves all dimensions of life and an integration of these dimensions within a unique being whose self continues to emerge. Holism implies also that the person is at peace with the surrounding environment. In this book the authors look at the older person achieving the high degree of integration and selfhood that Maslow calls self-actualization. From this discussion emerges a new respect for older people. Such a change in attitudes is one of the principal aims of nursing programs in relation to gerontology.

This book deals with assessment. In a very helpful way it takes theoretical formulations and applies them to the assessment step of the nursing process. Thus the student is helped to bring together the academic and clinical milieu.

Nursing students in baccalaureate programs will find this a most useful resource in holistically assessing healthy aged adults and in planning and providing wellness-oriented care.

Beryl H. Brubaker, R.N., M.S.
Assistant Professor
Department of Nursing
Eastern Mennonite College
Harrisonburg, Virginia

preface

The motivation for writing this book came from a need of nursing students enrolled in integrated health-oriented curricula. Well older people are often these students' first clients. Although many books are available about aging, geriatrics, and gerontology, the overwhelming theme in most of them is problems, illnesses, and the decline of the elderly.

This book focuses purposely on the "healthy" in an effort to give a clear picture of the well elderly person. The vast majority of older people are self-sufficient human beings who see themselves as healthy despite varying degrees of changes and losses. Promotion and maintenance of the healthy state is the goal of the nurse who relates to the well elderly client. Therefore, the focus of this book is on a holistic view of the well older person.

A human being, at any age, is a complex creature. Cultural, psychological, sociological, physical, spiritual, and environmental factors influence the development, the interests, and the activities of a person at any age. However, as humans age, they become increasingly more complex and integrated, often with deepening understanding of self in relationship to surrounding influences. Sometimes the analysis needed to present a holistic viewpoint of the older person results in compartmentalization without an ultimate synthesis. It is hoped that this is not the case in this book. This book deals with various factors that influence the person in his or her continuing development throughout life. A goal of this book is to overcome the problems of compartmentalization by maintaining a holistic approach throughout and by a unified application of the parts in the final chapter.

Cultural variables of aging will be surveyed. The resources and challenges of emotional and physical health will be examined. Social, religious, and economic factors that are important components of life will be reviewed since they influence the elderly person. A continuum construct will be used to demonstrate the diversity of the "normal" aging experience.

In the first chapter, aging is defined, statistics are reviewed, and the heterogeneous characteristics of the elderly population are discussed. A philosophical basis for holistic nursing and the goal of nursing is presented.

The second chapter focuses on cross-cultural similarities and differences in definitions and concepts of aging. Cultural factors that influence the status of the aged in a society, such as belief and value systems and social organization, are presented.

Chapter 3 provides an overview of biological theories of aging. The importance of a balance among rest, activity, and nutrition to health promotion is discussed. The normal physical changes that accompany aging and physical examination norms that differ from those of the younger adult are presented.

A developmental theory of aging is used to outline the content in Chapter 4. Psychological health is described, and the importance of client perceptions is discussed. Common misnomers for behavioral variations, intellectual abilities, and successful coping behaviors are examined. Information about the psychological aspects of religion is included.

Chapter 5 discusses the influences of retirement, social security, and various governmental resources. Housing and financial challenges with which the older person must deal are examined.

Chapter 6 suggests a technique that can be used to increase the nurse's awareness of the older client's social milieu. Social network theory is used as a basis for describing a healthy social situation of a person. The use of the person's social resources to maintain independence is discussed.

Chapter 7 brings the component parts together to demonstrate a holistic approach to client-centered nursing assessment and goal setting.

This book does not present an exhaustive study of the aging process. Readers who wish to pursue the components in more depth are encouraged to use the annotated bibliography and list of references along with other available resources.

There are many people in my social network who deserve acknowledgment for their contributions and support in the writing of this book. I want to especially thank the following people for their criticisms and suggestions about content accuracy, and clarity. From the University of Iowa: Leslie Marshall, Marjorie Price, Susan Uecker, Alberta Tedford, Geraldine Busse, Denise Ross, and Marie Faynor, all from the

College of Nursing; and John Menninger, Zoology; Gene F. Lata, Biochemistry; David Leslie, Physical Education; and Richard Horwitz, American Studies. Olive Wyse, Professor Emeritus of Home Economics at Goshen College, and Beryl H. Brubaker, Assistant Professor of Nursing at Eastern Mennonite College, also provided helpful advice. Also, I want to thank my efficient and patient typist, Jolene C. Klassen, for her fine work.

Miriam Martin Schrock, R.N., M.S.
Kalona, Iowa

contents

holistic assessment
of the
healthy aged

chapter one
a holistic view
of aging

Age creeps up so stealthily that it is often with shock that we become aware of its presence. Perhaps that is why so many of us reach old age utterly unprepared to meet its demands. We may be a bit rebellious about accepting it; I want to cry out that the invisible part of me is not old. . . .

A new set of faculties seems to be coming into operation. I seem to be awakening to a larger world of wonderment—to catch little glimpses of the immensity and diversity of creation. More than at any other time in my life, I seem to be aware of the beauties of our spinning planet and the sky above. And now I have the time to enjoy them. I feel that old age sharpens our awareness. . . .

Polly Francis, age 91
The Washington Post, March 16, 1975

OUTLINE

DEFINING AGING

Introduction

Defining aging is an herculean task, since different belief systems, societal norms, physical changes, and emotional responses contribute to a general lack of agreement on the meaning of aging and being old. Adding to the lack of clarity is the fact that neither research nor experience provides the data necessary for a universally satisfactory definition. Moreover, a holistic approach to aging and the aged can result in a seemingly superficial overview of the issue. Holism, as used here, is the concept that describes a person in his or her completeness as a being who is greater than the sum of his or her parts. Such a being can be partly understood through an objective evaluation of these parts, but such an understanding is incomplete without the perspective provided by the person's subjective evaluation of his or her own unity and uniqueness.

The ambiguity that exists in the absence of an acceptable definition of aging results in arbitrary decisions about when middle age ends and old age begins. A good example of such decisions is American society's arbitrarily determined laws and regulations, which state that retirement shall begin at the age of 65. This decision has resulted in a societal norm affecting everyone. Moreover, a person's definition and description of aging will greatly influence his or her perception of the age of 65 and retirement as a positive or negative experience.

Historically, humankind has always been interested in the aging process. The concern has, however, been more with preventing the process of aging than with accepting and understanding the process. Hippocrates and Aristotle saw aging as a natural phenomenon. Some people saw aging as a disease for which there was no cure. The ancient Chinese believed that aged people possessed supernatural abilities. During the Reformation, older citizens were accorded high status.

As America was being established as a nation in the seventeenth and eighteenth centuries, the aged were seen as people who were wise, experienced, and strong. When this country entered the industrial era, a variety of changes occurred and the aged decreased in importance, while youth became the admired segment of the population. This "youth cult" continues to be a factor of some importance in American culture.

With improvements of life-style and advancements in medical science during the twentieth century, greater numbers of people have lived longer, and aging has become more of a social problem than a social resource.

Definitions of Aging

A dictionary definition of aging states simply that aging is the process of growing mature or old. Alex Comfort in *A Good Age* divides the definition of aging into two components: biological and sociogenic aging. Biological aging refers to those physical changes, such as wrinkles and gray hair, that remind us of our mortality. On the other hand, sociogenic aging is "the role which society imposes on people as they reach a certain chronologic age" (1). Although many unanswered questions exist about the mechanisms of biological aging, the greatest source of questions and confusion about aging arises from the phenomenon of sociogenic aging.

Aging is still seen as a natural process, but often there are negative overtones to this concept. For example, aging is often portrayed as something one would escape if one had the power to do so.

A holistic definition of aging should communicate the idea that the changes associated with aging are normal and continuous, resulting in losses and gains. Even though the term "losses" evokes negative images, older people often experience change so gradually that they develop successful coping skills and accept the change as a normal part of life. An example of such an adaptation process would be a person's response to the pain that accompanies arthritis. Arthritis is a health problem often experienced as part of aging; however, the changes are gradual and a person usually finds ways to continue the activities he or she enjoys while accepting the discomfort as part of life. Moreover, the involvement in a pleasurable activity may be so great that the person forgets about the discomfort, at least temporarily.

The author chooses to define aging as a process of change during which a perspective is developed that brings wholeness to life while one gets older chronologically. Aging occurs on a continuum, and there are no discrete demarcations between adolescence, maturity, middlescence, and senescence. Proverbs that support this continuum idea are "you are as old as you feel" or "old is a state of mind." Even these sayings, which seem to counteract the idea of old age as a period of decline, continue a negative connotation for the term "old." A mind-set of senescence as a valued and beautiful period of life is not typical in America.

Regardless of how aging is defined, it is a salient topic for health professionals and the general public, since the aging process is experienced by everyone, and everyone who lives long enough will get old.

POPULATION STATISTICS ON AGING

A Changing Picture

Absolute statements about the size of the elderly population are somewhat unreliable because the numbers are continually changing. However, the United States Bureau of the Census is the best source of statistical information about population in America, and the statistics obtained from the United States Census, which are compiled every 10 years, are quite accurate. In addition, the population estimates and projections for the future are scientifically determined on the basis of demographic data such as the birth rate, immigration trends, and death rate.

Butler states that "every day, 1,000 people reach sixty-five" (2). It is evident from the population statistics that the over-65 category is continuously increasing (see Table 1). In the 60 years from 1870 to 1930, the percentage of the population over 65 years old changed only from 3

Table 1. Changes in the Aging Population in the United States

Year	Number of People over 65	Percentage of Population
1870	1,153,649	3
1900	3,080,498	4
1930	6,633,805	5
1950	12,269,537	8
1970	20,065,502	10
1980	24,910,000	11
2000	31,451,000	13
2020	43,425,000	16
2040	50,703,000	19

to 5%. This was during a time when the total population in the United States was increasing at a record rate. During the years 1930 to 1970, a span of only 40 years, the percentage of population over 65 doubled. During this time, the total population continued to increase at a remarkable rate (see Fig. 1) (3).

The decade since 1970 and the projections for the upcoming half century show a definite slowing in the rate of increase of the total United States population, while the percentage of the population over 65 is increasing at a more rapid rate than any time in history. Therefore, it is obvious that the needs of older people in our society are increasingly important both now and in the future (4, 5).

Life Expectancy and Life Span

It is helpful at this point to differentiate between the meaning of life expectancy and life span. *Life expectancy* is the statistic that describes the length of life of the average person. However, *life span* is the statistic that refers to the longevity of the most long-lived persons. Life-expectancy statistics relate to all causes of death at any age, so a decrease in infant mortality automatically increases this statistic but has no influence on life span data. Life span has not increased much over the centuries. Even the life span stated in the Bible is "seventy years—or eighty, if we have the strength" (Psalms 90:10). Thus, 70 or 80 years of life has been the expected longevity of long-lived persons for many years.

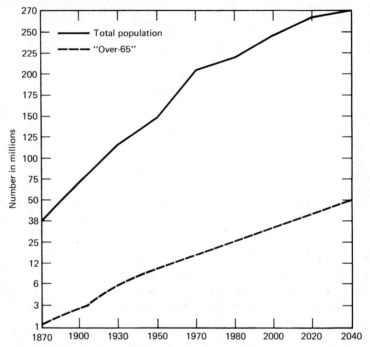

Figure 1. Total and Over-65 Population in the United States, 1870–2040.

Categories of Old Age

Even though the artibrary choice of 65 years as the beginning of old age is being challenged on legal and ethical grounds, changing that division point to 70 or 75 years would affect the elderly population statistics only minimally, since the number of people over 75 is increasing remarkably. Some gerontologists have divided old age into two categories: early old age (65 to 74 years) and advanced old age (above 75 years). However, the number of people over 85 years of age is also increasing. For this reason, a more precise division would be the one used by other gerontologists. These categories are: young old, old old, and very old (see Table 2).

As shown in Table 2, there has been a consistent increase in the over-75 and over-85 population, while the 65- to 74-year-old category is predicted to decrease gradually. In the next several decades it is predicted that there will be a remarkable increase in the 75-to-84 and the above-85 age groups.

As the older population in our society becomes numerically more

Table 2. Percentage of Aged Population in Three Categories of Old Age

	1900	*1950*	*1970*	*1975*	*1980*	*2000*	*2040*
Young-old (65 to 74 years)	71	69	62	62	62	55	48
Old-old (75 to 84 years)	25	27	31	30	29	33	37
Very old (over 85 years)	4	5	7	8	9	12	15

significant it is essential that we view this population holistically. Unfortunately, the very use of statistics to document the importance of older people in our society tends to compartmentalize and label rather than to provide a holistic approach. We will now view aging as a heterogeneous process.

THE HETEROGENEITY OF AGING

Normal aging can be described as having heterogeneous characteristics. The dictionary defines *heterogeneous* as "consisting of dissimilar constituents" (6). For well elderly persons, a variety of physiological and psychological coping skills have been developed during the years of life experience. Thus, the physiological and personality characteristics of old age span a broader range than in any other age group. Therefore, the range of "normal" characteristics is wide and can be described as heterogeneous, both for the individual and the group.

Each person has a broad range of coping mechanisms that he or she has found to be effective for him/herself. Moreover, the variation of effective coping behaviors can be multiplied by the number of people who have lived successfully into old age. The longer a person lives, the more numerous and varied are his or her life experiences. The challenges and triumphs of day-to-day living provide each person with inner resources, which increase his or her skill in coping with life. The result is often a rich storehouse of knowledge, emotion, and creativity that is beyond the scope of a person who has lived fewer years. Herein lies the wisdom that the old can share with the young—if the channels of communication are open.

Research data support the idea that heterogeneity among people increases with age. During a 40-year longitudinal study of 142 aging persons who lived in their own homes, data collected from the subjects were compared with data they had provided 40 years earlier when they were in the young- to middle-adult years. Components of the subjects' life-styles and personalities were compared. The range of responses was greater than in the earlier period of life. For example, some of the people who were satisfied with their marriage earlier in life responded that now marriage was better, others saw no change, and some perceived their marriage to be worse now. The study also found that most subjects were "psychologically well-functioning and healthy persons" (7).

Such research studies provide support for the belief of a growing number of people who work with the aging population that the aged are "not readily quantified or labeled" (8), and that old age does not always produce decline. Rather, "old age can provide a second and better chance at life" (7) and is a time when each person can integrate the many complexities of life more effectively.

The focus of this book is on the person who is aged; however, it is impossible to be holistic in approach without including the person's family. The family is usually defined as a group of people who are consanguineous or related by marriage, but the family also includes non-consanguineous members of the same household. The concept of *significant others* is sometimes used to denote more clearly an expanded nonconsanguineous view of family.

The status of families and individual persons in relation to various components of the whole can be visualized by use of the continuum construct. This is an especially helpful tool when one is describing the characteristics of a heterogeneous population. A *continuum* is defined as "something consisting of a series of variations or of a sequence of things in regular order" (6). A continuum can be used to picture the broad categories needed to see aging holistically. Such a tool is helpful, since discrete division points are hardly possible when dealing with a diversified population. However, the continuum is also helpful for placing a person at a specific point so his or her status and needs can be assessed accurately.

The normal distribution curve can be used in conjunction with the continuum construct to portray the distribution of the population within various categories. The normal distribution construct makes it easier to assess a specific person's status in relation to the larger population. It should be remembered that the use of these constructs constitutes a form of labelling or categorizing that should be used only as a tool. Examples of the combined use of the continuum and the normal distribution curve are shown in Figure 2.

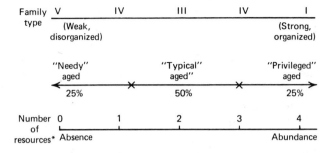

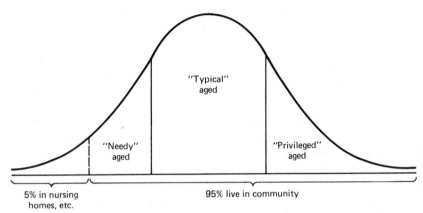

Figure 2. Use of continuum and normal distribution. Curve to describe the elderly population. (Adapted from date in Streib GF: Older families and their troubles: familial and social responses. *The Family Coordinator,* January 1972, pp. 5–19.)

A view of the human being as a developing, changing person who becomes more heterogeneous as he or she ages is based on a holistic philosophy of humankind.

A PHILOSOPHICAL BASIS FOR HOLISM

Historical Framework

The term *philosophy* comes from the Greek roots *philos* ("love") and *sophia* ("wisdom") and is defined as "a critical study of fundamental beliefs and grounds for them" (6). A review of traditional philosophies reveals an essential dichotomy.

As early as the time of Plato, Aristotle, and the Hebraic writers, humans have been seen in one of two ways: either as active or as passive beings. Historically, these viewpoints suggested two distinct and opposing interpretations of a person's involvement in shaping his or her own destiny. However, a holistic view of the basic character of the human implies that these two interpretations are not mutually exclusive, but can be seen as the extremes of a continuum, representing various degrees of belief about the determination of human destiny.

It is possible to extract portions of the writings of Plato and Aristotle to show that each of these philosophers upheld the concept of holism, even though they differed in the emphasis they placed on the physical world and its importance to human destiny. Plato focused on the beauty of goodness and order and rejected things that were merely physical. On the other hand, his student, Aristotle, although he viewed the universe as Plato did, focused on the unity of nature with goodness. He emphasized the importance of the human being's rational skills in understanding the physical world. Aristotle taught that through the use of the rational process, humans were striving to achieve completeness as persons. The Greek philosophers functioned in an environment of many gods; however, their gods were "surrounded by the sublime incomprehensibility of Fate, limiting their (the gods') knowledge and power" (9).

On the other hand, Hebraic philosophy was based on the power, love, and justice of one God. The monotheistic Hebrews saw God as being in charge of humankind's destiny, although they had a covenant relationship with their God. They recognized the human being's responsibility to live according to divine commands. In this, they acknowledged partial responsibility for their destiny. If they obeyed His commands, they experienced God's love and His power was at their disposal. If they chose not to obey, they incurred God's wrath. The Hebraic philosophy includes the human's rational response, which is absent in the ultimate fatalism of Greek philosophy. In other words, the way in which the Greeks responded to their gods had no influence on the ultimate behavior of Fate. Centuries later, St. Thomas Aquinas expanded Aristotelian philosophy to include the monotheistic God, whose reality was described by Saint Thomas as being greater than man's reality.

Various philosophical traditions have developed in the past 2,000 years and all have been influenced by both Greek and Hebrew philosophy. Efforts to systematize beliefs have produced numerous definitions, categorizations, and descriptions of the nature of humans. Often the efforts have provided documentation for a philosopher's position but, in so doing, have limited the search for holism.

A search for one philosophical tradition as a basis for holism is likely to end in frustration. Humanism comes close to holism, yet tends to underestimate the physical person. In addition, the subjective components of the human being, which humanists emphasize, are not easily categorized or measured. From a historical perspective, Hebraic philosophy can be considered to be the closest to holism. The commands of God in the Talmud are summarized by Jesus: "Hear, O Israel, the Lord our God, the Lord is one. Love the Lord your God with all your heart and with all your soul and with all your mind and with all your strength . . . and love your neighbor as yourself" (Mark 12:29–31). He speaks of the whole person: emotion, spirit, intellect, and body relating to God and his fellow human beings holistically, that is, "as yourself."

Both the humanistic and holistic approaches are judged to be too subjective by those who believe that only things that can be observed and rationally explained form an acceptable basis for philosophy. The frustration resulting from this schism is partly responsible for the development of existentialism, which was basically a revolt against the repudiation of traditional philosophy (9).

> Existentialism is not a system of philosophy; it can best be understood as an attitude or way of thinking. . . . Central to an understanding of existential thought is clarification of the concepts essence and existence. Essence, that which is, or the "I," refers to the nature of things; existence can be explained as the "am": I (a being) am (exist). The two are co-principles and must therefore be taken together. To think of nonexistent essences would tax our imagination almost as much as conceptualizing an existence without a supporting essence. There are, in fact, two components of man: his self or being, and the fact that he has continuance in life; that is, he exists from one minute to the next. The fact that man has being is called essence. The fact that man lives is called existence (10, p. 24).

Kaufmann (9) says that even though there is a great variety of opposing beliefs among existentialists "all of them contrast inauthentic life and authentic life." Ulsafer outlines three areas of general agreement among existentialists: 1) the worth of the person, 2) the person's free will (freedom to choose), and 3) a person's self-realization is best achieved through relationships with others (11).

Focus for Nursing

The complete answer to a philosophical methodology for the nursing profession is not an existential approach to philosophical thought. If the nursing profession's primary focus is on relating to people, then existential, humanistic, and idealistic philosophies seem adequate and appropriate. However, the effort to focus on science and scholarship in the nursing profession seems to call for objective, positivistic, and rationalistic philosophies (11). That nursing is not alone among the professions in this holistic versus particularistic dilemma does not decrease the importance of the issue for nursing. A synthesis of philosophical traditions that will result in a holistic philosophy appears to be necessary.

Moreover, the process of philosophical synthesis is a somewhat personal task for each nurse to engage in so he or she can find a unified perspective for practice. Psychological and social theories are sometimes helpful in such a synthesis. Social systems theory has made an effort to describe holism. Some ideas of social science that seem appropriate to the nursing profession are "the whole is more than the sum of the parts," "the parts cannot be understood if considered in isolation from the whole," and "the parts are dynamically interrelated or interdependent" (12). The analysis of a part provides information about the nature of the whole, but it does not provide enough information to describe the whole accurately. In nursing assessment, then, we can say that there is both a scientific and experiential basis for establishing assessment guidelines. Furthermore, these guidelines are tempered by the client's perception of his or her situation. Thus, the nurse comes to the client with his/her own knowledge and life experiences, seeking to understand the client's objective and subjective status.

When the client is elderly, he or she usually has a larger repertoire of life experience than does the nurse. The older person has usually gained and lost more in life than has a younger person. In addition, she or he is a reflection of a societal value system in relation to these life experiences.

Aging in American society is more often described in relation to losses than to gains. Many of the problems that have been identified with the process of aging can be categorized under loss of control over an aspect of life. Terms such as *depersonalization, loss of self-worth, helplessness, loss of purpose, decreased ability to function,* and *disengagement* are used to describe the aspects of the aging process that relate to losses. These terms are usually perceived as negative in character.

Much of what has been written about aging focuses on the losses the aging person experiences, with little discussion of gains, growth, and other descriptions that have positive connotations. Illness rather than the wellness of the aging person has been emphasized. Moreover, research has shown that the older person reflects the attitudes of society. Thus, when society as a whole has a basically negative attitude about the aging process and the status of being old, older people within that society are likely to have negative attitudes about themselves and to perceive themselves as not being in control of their own lives.

Ageism is a term coined by Dr. Robert Butler to describe society's attitude about aging. He defines ageism as "a process of systematic stereotyping of and discrimination against people because they are old" (2). The concept of ageism embodies, in part, what Alex Comfort refers to as sociogenic aging. Ageism is the phenomenon that results in the many labels applied to persons who are over 65.

When labels are imposed on members of a particular group within a society, it is evident that they are being viewed stereotypically, and either prejudice or the intent to dominate the group is operating. Terms that connote prejudice include *senior citizen, golden oldies,* or *sunset years* when referring to the group. When individual older persons are called Gramps, Pop, dearie, Grandma, sweetie, little old lady, and so on, they are being viewed stereotypically rather than individually.

Ageism tends to remove independence and self-direction from the citizens who have been leaders in family and community life for many years. Responses by the older person to these efforts ranges from complete resignation to militant resistance.

A holistic philosophy for the nursing profession can aid in combating ageism and in achieving nursing's goal of helping the client to assess his or her abilities and the solutions to the challenges he or she faces.

NURSING'S GOAL WITH THE WELL OLDER PERSON

Nursing's Primary Task

The nursing profession's primary task involves helping clients to cope with their perception of their experiences. A review of various definitions of nursing and descriptions of nursing practice through the years reveals that this basic goal of independent nursing practice has not changed remarkably. However, nursing terminology is becoming more systematic and scientific, and nursing is now described as a process. The components of the nursing process are assessment, planning, implementation of the plan, and evaluation of the effectiveness of the implementation. Nursing is an ongoing, interdependent process that, when carried out in its complete sense, includes the client on a continuous basis. Assessment, planning, implementation, and evaluation, if effective, are done jointly by client and nurse. The ultimate, if not the initial, goal is for the client to assume responsibility for his or her own care (13–15).

Client-Centered Assessment

When a thorough health or nursing assessment is made, the client can be placed at a point within a health/illness continuum. Holistic assessment involves evaluation of the client's cultural and environmental resources, his or her physical and emotional health, and his or her economic and social resources. A thorough assessment is best accomplished by full use of the three basic tools of assessment: *1)* general naturalistic observation, *2)* health history data, and *3)* a physical examination. At times the emphasis placed on the physical examination component of assessment results in overlooking significant data that could have been obtained by naturalistic observation and history taking.

When the nurse is involved in holistic assessment, complete interaction with the client is important in data collection. General naturalistic observations are initiated when the client first enters the nurse's field of vision. Does the client walk smoothly? Does he/she seem to be able to pick up auditory and visual cues from the immediate environment? Does he/she seem happy or sad? These questions are just a few examples of the kinds of thoughts the nurse should have when first observing the client. As an interaction with a client continues, it is important for the nurse to continue naturalistic observation, since verbal cues, which the client gives, may be important. The naturalistic observations that the nurse makes are often the basis for more specific questions during the history-taking component of the assessment process or for more detailed evaluation during a physical examination. For example, the client who limps when walking might be asked during the history-taking period what caused the limp, how long it has been present, and what effect it has on the client's life-style. During the examination, muscle strength and neurological status would be completely assessed.

There are many useful formats for the nursing history component of the assessment, and many nurses may wish to develop their own. However, for a client to be considered holistically, several things must be kept in mind. First, since the nurse seeks to help clients cope with their perceptions of their situations, ascertaining client perceptions of their present state of health is important. Does the client believe he/she is healthy? How is *healthy* defined? Has the client's state of health changed significantly in the recent past? Does the cultural group's definition of health influence the client's activity level or nutritional status? Do clients describe themselves as being satisfied with their life-style? Are they able to achieve most of the goals they establish? Third, do they believe their financial resources are adequate to meet their needs and wants?

Nursing assessment provides a joint assessment in that the client's abilities are listed along with his or her challenges in the nursing diagnosis, the end product of nursing assessment (15). When the assessment is undertaken jointly, the nurse and client can agree on a plan to deal with the challenges that have been identified, which can be implemented under the direction of the client.

After the nursing diagnosis is made, the goal of nursing intervention is to help increase the client's resources or to find new ones. Interventions vary in response to each particular challenge. However, some common areas that involve the mutual efforts of the nurse and client include nutritional status, exercise and activity, and socialization. An underlying goal of nursing intervention with the elderly client is to help dispel myths so the client and his or her family can use creative, self-directed approaches to achieve a meaningful life-style.

The Ethic of the Right to Self-Determination

A view of nursing intervention based on a holistic, synthesized philosophy is congruent with the ethic that each person has a right to self-determination. In our social system, social leaders and citizens who are in charge of much of what happens have this right to self-determination. Conversely, the people who are, by the labels applied to them, classified as dependent (children, adolescents, and senior citizens) do not have this right. Therefore, a holistic philosophical stance for nursing in relation to the elderly provides a guideline for returning the right of self-determination to older people. The belief that older people have the right of self-determination is consistent with the fact that the older person's life experiences and resulting wisdom give him or her intrinsic resources to cope with a broad spectrum of challenges.

SUMMARY

The healthy aged comprise a significant portion of the population for whom the nursing profession provides its unique skills of holistic assessment and intervention. A philosophical base that is primarily holistic provides the nursing profession with a framework for relating to clients in a way that allows clients to remain in control of their own lives and life-styles. Nursing has an important role in assisting clients in the identification of their resources and challenges so their needs can be met in a manner congruent with the clients' perception of their own experiences.

REFERENCES

1. Comfort A: *A Good Age*. New York, Crown Publishers, 1976, p 9.
2. Butler RN: *Why Survive? Being Old in America*. New York, Harper & Row, Publishers, 1975, p 16.
3. US Bureau of the Census: *Historical Statistic of the United States, Colonial Times to 1970, Bicentennial Edition, Part 2*. Washington, DC, US Government Printing Office, 1975.
4. US Bureau of the Census: Projections of the population of the United States: 1977-2050. *Current Population Reports,* Series P-25, No. 704. Washington DC, US Government Printing Office, 1977.
5. US Bureau of the Census: Estimates of the population of the United States by age, sex and race: 1970–1977. *Current Population Reports,* Series P-25, No. 721. Washington, DC, US Government Printing Office, 1978.
6. *Webster's Third New International Dictionary.*
7. Mass HS, Kuypers JA: *From Thirty to Seventy*. San Francisco, Jossey-Bass Publishers, 1974, p 200.
8. National Institute on Aging: *Our Future Selves, A Research Plan Toward Understanding Aging* (DHEW Publication No. 77-1096). Washington, DC, Department of Health, Education and Welfare, 1977, p 20.
9. Kaufmann W: *Existentialism: From Dostoevsky to Sartre*. Cleveland, Ohio, The World Publishing Company, 1956.
10. Ulsafer J: A relationship of existential philosophy to psychiatric nursing. *Perspect Psychiatr Care* 14:23–28, 1976.
11. Zbilut JP: Epistemologic constraints to the development of a theory of nursing. *Nursing Res* 27:128–129, 1978.
12 Phillips DC: *Holistic Thought in Social Science*. Stanford, Calif, Stanford University Press, 1976, p 6.
13. Wiedenbach E: *Clinical Nursing A Helping Art*. New York: Spring Publishing Company, 1964.
14. Henderson V: The nature of nursing. *Am J Nurs* 64:62–68, 1964.
15. Little DE, Carnevali DL: *Nursing Care Planning,* ed 2. Philadelphia, JB Lippincott Company, 1976, pp 82–94.

ANNOTATED BIBLIOGRAPHY

Butler, RN: *Why Survive? Being Old in America.* New York, Harper & Row, Publishers, 1975.
A challenging book by a well-known psychiatrist/gerontologist that exposes the myths of aging and the vagrancies of societal responses to the aged and their needs and provides some alternative approaches to aging in America. Contains valuable appendices of literature and organizational and governmental resources for the elderly.

Comfort, A: *A Good Age.* New York, Crown Publishers, 1976.
A readable collection of explanations of the issues faced in aging that emphasizes the achievements of aging and the aged. Numerous examples are given of well-known people who have aged successfully.
Dr. Comfort is a leading, internationally known gerontologist whose research on the aging process during the past several decades has expanded the knowledge base in the field of aging.

deBeauvior, S: *The Coming of Age.* New York, G.P. Putnam's Sons, 1972. First published in Paris under title: *La Vieillesse,* 1970.
A historical view of the treatment of old people in the Western World. Explores myths used by various groups to idealize aging while old age is treated as a "shameful secret." Shows that a millenium of western civilization has not resulted in a unified positive response to the question "Are the old really human beings?"

McLeish, JA: *The Ulyssean Adult—Creativity in the Middle and Later Years.* Toronto, McGraw-Hill Ryerson, 1976.
The author uses various life-cycle theories as a background for extensive discussion and provides examples of productive, creative, joyful living in the second half of life.

chapter two
cultural perspectives on aging

We are not permitted to choose the frame of our destiny. But what we put into it is ours.

Dag Hammarskjöld

OUTLINE

CONTROVERSIES IN TRANSCULTURAL GERONTOLOGY
  Is the Status of the Aged Inversely Proportional to the Degree of
    Modernization?
  Is Disengagement a Cultural Universal?
  Do the Aged Comprise a Subculture in the United States?
IMPLICATIONS OF THE CULTURAL PERSPECTIVE FOR
  GERONTOLOGICAL NURSING
SUMMARY

Patterns of aging vary dramatically across different cultures. These divergent patterns pertain not only to the status and treatment of the elderly but also to biological aspects of aging, such as differences in life spans and degrees of physical and mental deterioration. Fuller (1) reported that marked senility is rare among the Bantu of South Africa. Leaf (2) and Alikishiyev (3) found high proportions (sometimes over 10%) of the total population to be above age 100 and life spans exceeding 150 years among such diverse groups as the Vilcabamba in Ecuador, the Hunza in West Pakistan and the Georgians in the Soviet Caucasus. These differences in biological variation have been attributed to many causes, including genetic composition, nutrition, physical activity, and social role responsibilities.

Aging is both a biological and a social process, and it must ultimately be understood from an integrated, multidisciplinary viewpoint. However, although a holistic orientation is necessary for understanding the aging process clearly, the initial focus of this chapter is on the relationships between patterns of aging and sociocultural factors. In examining the cultural dimension of aging, the following areas are considered: first, how aging is defined differently in various cultures; second, the variations in the status and treatment of the elderly; and third, controversies about theories pertaining to cultural patterns of aging.

UNIVERSALITY OF AGE CLASSIFICATION

After surveying the phenomenon of aging in a variety of societies ranging from preliterate to complex industrial, Cowgill and Holmes (4) concluded that just as all societies have systems of classifying persons according to sex and kinship, they also have a system that classifies people by age. One aspect of this age grading is that in all societies some people are considered "old." Furthermore, each society ascribes differential statuses and norms of behavior in terms of this classification, that is, the elderly are expected to behave and to be treated differently from people in other age classes within the society.

There are three general systems of age-group classification, which may be arranged along a continuum from least to most structured: *1)* the ordinal, *2)* the developmental life-crises, and *3)* the age-grade systems of classification.

Ordinal Classification

The ordinal classification system is based on the chronological age of participants. It indicates whether a person is older or younger than another person. In some societies, this differential relative age is the basis for determining relative social status; almost always the senior person is treated with deference, as indicated by language, avoidance, or other behavioral patterns.

Developmental Classification

The developmental classification system varies across cultures depending on which stages each society recognizes. These stages vary across time within a single society, as well as across different societies. For many years Western society did not recognize a period called "adolescence," and most recently, middlescence has been "discovered". Similarly, other cultures recognize periods of life crises and organize age classification systems according to these critical times. Among the Sidamo of southwest Ethiopia the periods of life crises for males include birth, early childhood, initiation, marriage, elderhood, exalted old age, and death (5).

Age-Grade Classification

The most structured system of classification is that of the age-grade. The term *age-grade* refers to a *social category* of people (usually of the same sex) who fall within the same culturally defined age range. These categories of age-grades form a series of graduated steps.

The term *age-set,* on the other hand, is used to describe the group of people who are initiated together into an age-grade. People of the same age group are initiated into the first age-grade when they are roughly the same chronological age. After a culturally specified number of years, a new age group is initiated into that age-grade, and the former occupants are initiated into the next higher age-grade. An age-set will move together through all of the age-grade categories.

Age-graded systems of classification are commonly found in African tribal societies. Figure 3 diagrams the age-grade system among the Masai, an East African cattle-herding society. During adolescence, boys undergo an initiation into the first age-grade. Throughout their lifetimes, members of this age-set who were initiated together into this first age-grade will move together to progressively higher age-grade categories.

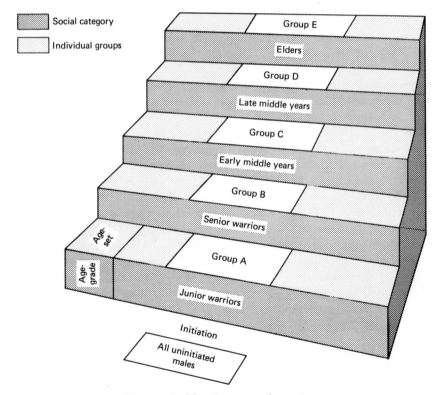

Figure 3. Masai age-grade system.

DEFINING THE AGED

All human societies use systems of age classification either singly or in combination, and differential roles and statuses are ascribed to people in these different age classes. Furthermore, in all societies, some people are considered to be "old," and, because of this designation, they are expected to behave and to be treated differently than people in other age categories.

However, the age at which a person enters the "old" category varies widely among different cultures. Clark and Anderson (6) noted that among the Maricopa Indians of Arizona, the term *old man* or *old woman* may be applied to a person in his early 40s. Mead (7) remarked that the Chinese entered the "honorable age" between 45 and 50 years. In Samoa, old age begins at age 50, when men are referred to as "old men"; then, sometime between the ages of 60 and 70, an additional name may be added, which would mean "very aged man" (8). In Thai society, age is computed in 12-year cycles, and old age begins on the sixtieth birthday, or at the completion of the fifth cycle (9). In Western societies, old age is generally thought to be begin when one retires from an active work life (between 65 and 70 years). Thus, the absolute chronological age at which people are considered to be "elderly" varies widely across cultures.

Interestingly, the elderly may not always accept the general societal standard. Regarding the age at which people consider themselves to be "old," Shanas (10) found that most people in the United States have a weak old age identification until they reach the age of 75; she found that 17% of the men in the United States in the 80 to 84 cohort still considered themselves as middle aged.

In part, these differences in the age at which people are considered "old" result because of the variety of general criteria used by societies for determining who is aged. Persons can be placed in age classes along several dimensions, which may be divided into four major groups: physical, functional, symbolic, or temporal criteria. These groups of criteria will be discussed separately, although they may exist singly or in combination in various societies.

Physical Criteria

Occasionally, a society will base the criteria for "elderly" solely on the manifestation of certain physical traits. In New Guinea, Kapuku men and women are considered "old" when their hair becomes gray (11).

Dentan (12) also found that among the Semai of Malaya a woman is considered to be an "oldster" when she has wrinkled breasts and white hair. More often, however, societies use physical appearance in combination with other criteria.

Functional Criteria

In some societies, people are determined to be "old" when they can no longer carry out their adult role functions. Functional criteria, then, are based on the degree of physical and/or mental deterioration. Shelton (13) found among the Sidamo of southwest Ethiopia that people are considered to be aged by the time they are chiefly the recipients rather than the furnishers of goods and services. The Siuai are considered to be old when they become so senile that the soul is thought to leave the body more often than it is present (14), and some Malayans are considered "old" when they have but can no longer bear children (12).

Symbolic Criteria

A person may be defined as aged after the occurrence of some socially symbolic event. This criterion has a particularly wide range of variation because culturally significant symbols differ vastly. Among the Maricopa Indians of Arizona, a person is considered "old" if he or she has a grandchild (6). Fuller (1) found that among the Bantu of South Africa, one assumes the role of elder on the death of the senior males of one's lineage. In Samoa, a man is held to be "old" when he assumes the head position in an extended family, regardless of his chronological age (8).

Temporal Criteria

Temporal criteria may be based on actual chronological age or, as with the case of age-graded societies, the chronology of one's age-set. While age classification based on temporal criteria is not restricted to Western societies, with their highly amplified methods of time and record keeping, it is most elaborate in these societies.

There are, however, differences in the manner in which chronological age is calculated. The Chinese (among others) compute age from the assumed time of conception; in Western societies age is calculated from the time of actual birth. Furthermore, as previously noted, the exact chronological age when a person is considered "old" may range from the mid-40s to 70.

Thus, we find that there are a number of different methods of assessing and ascribing age in various cultures. The salient points about aging criteria are *1*) in each society, there is at least one method for ascribing status and roles based on an age classification system; *2*) some people in all societies are considered "old"; and *3*) the Western system of classification is only one of a number of possible methods.

TRANSCULTURAL VARIATIONS IN STATUS AND TREATMENT OF THE AGED

Range of Variation

Just as there is no universal method of classifying the elderly, there are also no universals about the status and treatment of the aged. While all societies define a certain group as elderly, there is a wide variation in the way members of the society perceive the aged person; the aged as a group may be highly regarded or largely disvalued. In some societies old age is a time of high prestige and power, while in others it is a time of insecurity and alienation. Old age may be the time when people enjoy the greatest respect or when they must endure psychological or physical abandonment.

In the United States the aged are typically stereotyped as unproductive, physically and mentally deteriorated, poverty stricken, disengaged, and burdensome. However, this middle-class American stereotype is only one of a number of possible ways in which the aged may be viewed by a society. As Palmore noted, we may be unaware that in other cultures the aged are the most powerful, the most engaged, and the most respected members of the society (15).

Although we can make generalizations about the status of the aged in certain "types" of societies, (e.g., respect for the elderly is more often higher in slowly changing societies), such generalizations actually tell us very little about the social basis for this heightened prestige; they only correlate a fact with a type. We need to investigate in greater depth the social reasons for the cross-cultural variations in status, roles, and treatment of the aged.

Status and role changes occur in all societies across the life cycle. As a general rule, the status of the aged decreases with increased modernization and technological complexity. That is, the status of the aged is generally highest in hunting/gathering and agricultural (peasant) societies and lowest in technologically complex, industrialized societies. However, this generalization is only useful as a heuristic tool.

Regarding the social basis for prestige, Simmons (16) noted that respect for old age results from social discipline. In indigenous societies, there are no signs of a deep-seated instinct to guarantee to elders either homage or pity from their offspring. Whatever prestige they receive is not a natural phenomenon; it is a product of social developments.

Factors Influencing Status and Treatment

A number of factors influence the way in which the aged are perceived and treated in any given society. These factors can be grouped into four main categories: *1)* value systems; *2)* belief systems; *3)* social structural components (including economic, kinship, political, and religious configurations), and *4)* suprasystem factors (such as ecology and rate of culture change), which are closely interrelated to the operations and mechanisms of the other three categories.

These factors are diagrammed in Figure 4. Although these elements are arranged in a hierarchy, the direction of influence is not only unidirectional. Although values underly our beliefs and attitudes, they

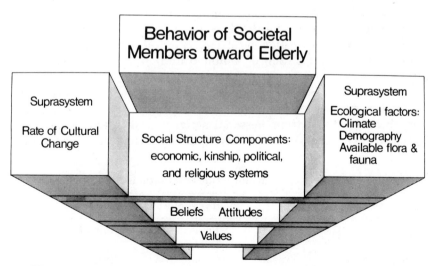

Figure 4. Factors influencing status and treatment of the elderly.

can be inferred only indirectly from our behaviors. In addition, the separation of these factors is only for ease of discussion, for in any social system these elements are continuously interacting and forming a mutually reinforcing feedback system.

Value Systems

In a discussion of the influences that cause variations in the status and the treatment of the aged, those elements that pattern the behaviors of the societal members must first be considered. These factors, which set the rules of living, are values, beliefs, and attitudes. In discussing concomitants of status, the initial emphasis should be on value orientations because they are the most basic of all cultural normative systems.

Values may be considered as ordering mechanisms that provide the basis for attitudes and behaviors of a group of people, and as noted by King (17) values tell us how to choose among objects and events and how to establish hierarchies of needs and goals. Values usually operate on an unconscious level, and their presence usually can be inferred only through analysis of behavior.

Kluckhohn and Strodbeck (18) devised a paradigm of dominant value orientations that presents the various ways in which a social group may choose to perceive and to order certain human problems. Value orientations are "complex but definitely patterned (rank-ordered) principles, resulting from the transactional interplay of three analytically distinguishable elements of the evaluative process—the cognitive, the affective, and the directive elements—which give order and direction to the ever-flowing stream of human acts and thoughts as these relate to the solution of 'common human' problems" (18, p.4). Table 3 is a modified version of their paradigm.

Kluckhohn and Strodbeck organized various problems with which all societies must cope. They considered the way that humans organize their thinking about time, personal activity, and interpersonal relations. Here is an analysis of the ways these variations in value orienta-

Table 3. Dominant and Variant Value Orientations

Orientation	Range of Variations		
Time	Past	Present	Future
Activity	Being	Doing	
Relational	Lineal	Collateral	Individualistic

tions influence the status and treatment of the aged in different cultures.

Time Orientation.   The temporal orientation may be broken into three dimensions: past, present and future.

Past: Historical prerevolutionary China is an example of a society where "past" time orientation is given dominence. "Ancestor worship and a strong family tradition were both expressions of this preference. So also was the Chinese attitude that nothing new ever happened in the Present or would happen in the Future; it had all happened before in the far distant past" (18, p.14).

In oriental cultures, past services or outstanding accomplishments of elders are more likely to be remembered as unpaid obligations by younger societal members.

Present: Traditional European peasant societies may be characterized as being oriented toward the present. Here the future is regarded as both vague and unpredictable. Primary concern lies with problems of the present: droughts, floods, planting, and harvesting.

Future: A futuristic orientation is characteristic of modern highly technological societies such as American middle-class culture. In American society, we are most concerned with progress and the planning for the future. With built-in obsolescence, new is better than old, whether the topic is thinking, products, or people. This future-oriented approach moves us inexorably away from the past. The aged in a future-oriented society are not valued because they do not assist in progress and will not participate in the future.

In summary, societies with orientations toward the past or present tend to grant the aged higher status than do societies with an orientation toward the future.

Activity Orientation.   The activity orientation discerns whether a given culture is primarily ordered toward a doing (or achievement) mode of action or a being mode.

Being: In societies with a being orientation, each person is valued for his or her very existence (not for his or her accomplishments). This pattern is typical of corporate-lineage groups, in which the person is valued as a link in a chain of continuity between generations. The Igbos of Nigeria, described by Shelton (13, 19), typify this orientation. Furthermore, here as in other such societies, the dependency of the aged on the food-producing adults has positive acceptance. The Igbo is dependent on the gods, the ancestors, the elders, and the lineage itself; reciprocal dependence is acknowledged. A child living in Igbo society is no more dependent than his elders, he is simply dependent on different things.

Thus, the dependency that accompanies very old age is not something to be rejected but to be valued. As Simmons noted, "With vitality declining, the aged person has had to rely more and more upon personal relations with others, and upon the reciprocal rights and obligations involved" (16). In societies where these social relations are most formalized, the aged can make the transition to a dependent position more easily.

Doing: The middle-class American has been characterized as "doing," that is, as having an achievement mode of activity. Each person is valued for his or her accomplishments, not for his or her inherent existence. Mainstream American culture has tended to stress the importance of work and competition. The retirement of the mainstream American from a highly competitive, work-oriented life-style into one with fewer visible achievements causes a decrease in self-esteem and social status. In addition, the dependency of the old who are no longer productively engaged in valued "doing" also tends to decrease the status of the aged in American society.

Thus, the elderly who live in societies in which the "being" orientation is dominant are less likely to be downgraded in status on arriving at the category of "old" than are the elderly in societies where each person is valued for what he or she is doing, not simply for his or her existence.

Relational Orientation. This orientation distinguishes among interpersonal patterns and is concerned with the ways in which the society, in general, sets goals for its individual members.

Collateral: When the collateral principle is dominant, the goals and welfare of the laterally extended group (sibs or members of the same age-set) are of prime importance. Collectivist societies typically demonstrate a collateral orientation. In both Russia (20) and Israel (21) the individual member is subordinated to group goals; but at the same time, the group maintains responsibility for all its members, including the elderly. The collateral principle is also frequently dominant among hunter/gatherers and herders. It may be most strikingly elaborated among the age-graded societies such as the previously mentioned Masai. In societies with a collateral relational orientation, each person's goals, security, and social value are not separable from those of the larger group.

Lineal: As with collateral orientation, when the lineal principle is dominant, group goals and group welfare have primary importance.

However, with the lineal orientation one of the important goals is continuity through time. Continuity of the group and ordered positional succession within the group are both crucial issues when lineality dominates.

In nearly all societies with an emphasis on lineality, kinship is the basis for maintaining the lineage. Most often, the group traces its descent through the male line, with authority resting with the eldest male or a male ancestor. In prerevolutionary China the lineage was the primary social-ordering mechanism (22, 23). The lineage fulfilled the functions of education, economic production, discipline, religion, and social programs (caring for the destitute, old, and infirm). In this clan society, filial piety was more important than spouse relationships or individualism, and the official leader of the lineage was the eldest living man.

Shelton (19) has demonstrated how the values of interdependence are instilled in the young in a lineage society. Among the Igbo of Nigeria, interdependence among the members of the community despite age differences are stressed by: *1)* de-emphasizing narrow or selfish individualism that could weaken the bonds of interdependence and *2)* showing that all age groups in the society are rewarded for their loyalty to the network of mutual rights and duties.

Thus, in lineal societies, the aged are often the most powerful members of the society. At the very least, they are well cared for because of their membership in the lineage.

Individualistic: When the individualistic principle is dominant, individual goals have primacy over the goals of specific collateral or lineal groups. Each person's responsibility to the total society and his place in it are defined by autonomous goals. Mainstream America, as well as most other industrialized Western societies, emphasizes the individualistic orientation. The person alone is held responsible for his/her behavior, and he/she alone is judged on the basis of his/her work. Religion is largely a personal matter (rather than a structured group experience), and work is not closely tied to the extended family.

In these individualistically oriented societies, when the aged members can no longer meet all their goals, they must be assisted by others, and this pattern is not congruent with their value system.

The individualistic orientation of Western societies promotes the alienation of the elderly, while lineal and collateral societies more adequately provide for the economic and also the psychological needs of the aged. Thus, societies with value systems that emphasize the collateral or lineal principle submerge the individual person in the group and provide more security for their members than do individualistically oriented societies, which place an emphasis on personal goals and achievements.

American Variations in Value Orientation. The United States contains diverse ethnic populations and thus exhibits greater heteroegeneity among older people than most other Western cultures.

Because it is ethnically diverse, the United States does not exhibit a uniform dominant value system. While a dominant value system can be identified for middle-class Americans, members of American subcultural groups may have dominant value orientations that vary considerably from those of mainstream America. An example of this and its importance for understanding the status and treatment of the aged can be found in the study by Clark and Mendelson of the aged in San Francisco (24). A summary of their results and a comparison of the dominant value orientation of the Anglo with that of the traditional Ladino aged in San Francisco is seen in Table 4.

In studying these two groups Clark and Mendelson found that the aged in the Anglo subculture were less well adapted and had lower levels of self-esteem than did the aged in the Ladino subculture. The Anglos based their self-evaluation on the criteria that were consistent with their dominant value orientations: achievement and success, aggressiveness, acquisition, activity and work, individualism, control, progress, and an orientation toward the future. Ladinos, on the other hand, based their self-esteem on a contrasting profile: they valued congeniality, reliance, harmoniousness, cooperation, continuity, and a present orientation.

Thus, the ways in which the aged within a subculture view themselves and are viewed and treated by other members of that subculture vary widely among different groups within the United States.

Belief Systems

In societies in which ancestor worship is practiced, as among many of the traditional Oriental cultures, the aged are generally accorded high status. Here, the aged person is the closest living relative to the revered ancestors, and as such, he or she maintains a highly revered position; he or she is the family member who will soon be joining the ancestors.

In societies with belief in spiritual ancestors, there is usually the corollary belief that these spirits can be either beneficial or harmful to the living. The aged are treated with great respect in these societies so when they become spirits, they will do good works and not harm to the family (13, 19).

Table 4. Anglo and Ladino Dominant Value Orientation

Orientation	Middle-Class Anglo	Ladino
Time	Future	Present
Activity	Doing (achievement)	Being
Interpersonal (relational)	Individualistic	Lineal-collateral
Man to nature	Dominant	Subjugated

In addition, in the majority of societies with belief in intervening spiritual ancestors, the lineage or clan elders are usually the intermediaries between the ancestoral world and the world of the living. Among the Nigerian Igbo the ancestors are thought to control fertility, illness, and death. The lineage elder is the person who is able to influence these ancestral spirits. Thus, the aged gain prestige from their proximity to the ancestors and from their ability to influence them.

In societies in which such a complex, well-delineated system of belief in an afterlife does not exist, death may be feared or considered a tragedy. For many Americans, the aged are viewed with apprehension because they are reminders of our mortality, rather than an extension of life into the spiritual world.

In cultures in which there is a belief in magical manipulations or sorcery, the idea that the aged control more ritual or secret knowledge necessary for curing or safety is often prevalent. The aged are respected because, by virtue of their successful living, they are evidence of having powerful knowledge and/or ritual powers. Among the Yahgans of South America nearly every old man was considered a wizard, and occasionally so were aged women (16); they inspired sufficient fear and respect to be treated well. The Labrador Eskimo treated the aged with great deference and regarded their words as final because it was believed that in them was embodied the wisdom of the ancestors. Old women were respected for their ability to interpret dreams, and aged men were renowned as healers (16).

Through the mechanism of secret societies, the aged may guard this sacred or ritual knowledge. Among the Druze, a religious sect in the Middle East, the aged traditionally keep the religion secret from the women and the younger men of the community (25).

Some belief systems promote an elevated status of the aged based on the symbolic meaning of age. Palmore (15) reports that among the Palaung in northern Burma, the aged enjoyed high prestige because long life was considered a great privilege, indicating virtuous behavior in a previous existence. In addition, in Bali the children and the very old have increased status because of their presumed proximity to heaven.

Finally, religious beliefs or writings may prescribe certain behavior toward the elders. Plath (26) reports that for more than 1,000 years, the Japanese have been exhorted to follow Confucian principles that demand honor and succor for elders in general and parents in particular. Streib (27) also reports that the basic Judeo-Christian tradition to honor one's father and mother is strongly instilled in the minds of the Irish. Here, traditional religion is important as a source and as a means of reinforcing reverence for the old.

Palmore (15) noted that among the three primary religious groups in American society, Jews appear to show the most respect and responsibility for their aged. Christianity developed in a Greco-Roman setting and was influenced by the Germanic culture, neither of which highly regarded its aged. Thus, Christians seem to have less respect and fewer feelings of responsibility for their aged than do Jews. Palmore also found that a greater range of attitudes toward the aged exists among Protestants than among Roman Catholics. Protestants more often tend to consider misfortune and failure as a result of moral insufficiency or a lack of responsibility and planning. Therefore, Protestants are often less sympathetic toward the misfortunes of their aged than are Roman Catholics or Jews.

Social Organization

While many authors often make the generalization that the status of the aged is higher in simpler societies, generalizing obscures the social basis for this tendency. In the manner of Mauss, who hypothesized that reciprocity is the foundation of social interaction, Simmons (16) found that increased status of the aged was tied to the degree to which they were able to perform valued functions in the society. In simpler societies, a number of factors tend to elevate the status of the aged. At times, these factors may operate singly, for example, high status may be achieved on the basis of one primary factor such as healing ability or land ownership; but more often, status results from a combination of these factors, each of which may have its origin in a different component of social organization.

In simpler societies, the components of social organization (kinship, economic, political, religious, and health systems) are closely interrelated, and they may not be perceived as separate systems by members of that society. In a society with corporate-lineage groups, which rely heavily on the elders for leadership, the elders may approach the ancestors for help and assistance in planting the crops, curing illness, making political decisions, and performing religious ceremonies. In these societies the family is the organizing unit, not a separate aspect, of society, and the aged are often the leaders. However, for the sake of clarity these dimensions of social organization will be discussed separately.

In this section, technoeconomic systems are given primary importance because this component of social organization is often basic to the development of other organizational components such as the political or kinship system. In addition, social factors directly associated with the level of technoeconomic development most clearly relate to the status and treatment of the aged. However, the purpose of the discussion is not to promote the notion of technoeconomic determinism, since cultural configurations and cultural change cannot be understood from a simple, unifactorial perspective.

TechnoEconomic Systems. Systems of economic production may be classified as hunting and gathering (including fishing), herding, horticultural, peasant agricultural, or industrialized. Without espousing the doctrines of economic or technological determinism, some generalities can be drawn about societies at different levels of technological development, because many social correlates are associated with particular technological levels. However, it must be pointed out that these are generalities and are not applicable to every society that is at a specific technological level.

After studying a range of cultural types, Cowgill and Holmes (4) concluded that role expectations for the aged always differ from those of younger people in all types of societies. Generally, the aged are graduated to less strenuous and less physically exacting pursuits. Even if there is not formal retirement, the old men are not expected to continue economic pursuits; they are commonly promoted to the positions of elder headman or priest. Thus, the aged shift from roles requiring high physical exertion to sedentary, advisory positions.

Hunting and gathering societies: Hunting and gathering was the first mode of production in the history of the human species. Although it was once universal, socioeconomic systems based on hunting and gathering are now found only in fringe areas of the world, where more technologically advanced forms of production are not feasible (e.g., in the ice-ridden areas of the north, in desert lands, and in rain forests).

Generally, in hunting and gathering societies the aged are encouraged to engage in any physical activity of which they are capable. Both aged men and women continue to perform their regular economic tasks until they are no longer physically able to do so. However, with the advent of physical or mental disabilities, there is some shift in the camp tasks these people will perform. The shift may occur first in the degree and finally in the type of work performed.

Watanabe (29) found that in many northern hunting groups there is a division of labor between adults and elderly; the younger men exploit more distant hunting areas and the older men hunt and fish nearer to the base camp. In addition, there are age differences in certain occupations; the younger men may spear fish while the older men ice fish; the young may hunt game, the old may butcher the kill. Thus, elders are differentiated in their work role, not only by a decreased geographic area but also by engaging in the less strenuous aspects of the particular economic activity.

A second form of age-role adaptation in hunting and gathering societies is a change in the sphere of activities for the elderly. Simmons (16) found that an important means by which the aged achieve security for themselves is to assist in the interests and enterprises of others. Older people in this group often adapt secondary economic roles and make themselves as useful as possible in the camps and households. For example, aged women among the Labrador Eskimo received food in exchange for the care of the men's boots and for other services.

Thus, in large measure, the aged in hunting and gathering societies are encouraged to function at valued tasks and to contribute to the economic sphere even after they demonstrate considerable physical deterioration.

What happens to the aged when they no longer are physically able to contribute in a hunting and gathering society is a matter of dispute. Turnbull, in speaking of the Mabuti pygmies living in the Ituri Forest in the Congo, noted:

> . . . old and infirm people are regarded . . . with apprehension. In a vigorous community of this kind, where mobility is essential, cripples and infirm people can be a great handicap and may even endanger the safety of the group. Hence there are numerous legends of old people being left to die if they cannot keep up with the group as it moves from camp to camp. . . . Sau knew this, and although she was still healthy she made sure everyone knew it by taking the most vigorous and unexpected part in any dispute, her sharp, acid voice betraying a certain bitterness at the way she was treated . . . (30, pp.35–36).

On the other hand, Richard Lee found a different pattern among the Bushmen of the African Kalahari Desert.

The aged hold a respected position in Bushman society and are the effective leaders of the camps. Senilicide is extremely rare. Long after their productive years have passed, the old people are fed and cared for by their children and grandchildren. The blind, the senile and the crippled are respected for the special ritual and technical skill they possess. For instance, the four elders at !Gose waterhole were totally or partially blind, but this handicap did not prevent their active participation in decision making and ritual curing (31, p.36).

Horticultural/Agricultural Societies: With the advent of plant and animal domestication came herding, horticulture, and, finally, agriculture. Simmons (16) hypothesized that it is in these middle-range societies that the aged obtain the highest status. A number of factors contribute to the high status of the elderly in these societies.

First, a new dimension enters the economic sphere as the base of economic activity shifts from the realm of physical power in hunting and fishing to the realm of jural control of property rights. Because hunting and gathering societies are usually quite mobile, there is little personal property; furthermore, rights to all the available lands and water areas are generally open to the entire band.

Although the aged in middle-range societies, like the elderly in other types of societies, lose the physical strength they had in their youth, they often maintain control over most aspects of property. The aged may either own the land or control its use allocation; this control is institutionalized through inheritance patterns or religious prescription.

Old men of the Chukchi receive great consideration, especially in the reindeer-breeding section of the tribe, because the herd belongs to the father as long as he lives. These men (perhaps 70 to 80 years old) have retained possession of the herd and have controlled the general direction of the life in their camps. Likewise, among the Akamba in Africa, the old men own all the cattle and the goats and none of their sons possess anything; even the sons' wives are bought with the elder's property. In turn, the dowry, as well as blood money, is used to increase the herds of the aged leader (16).

Therefore, we see that in agricultural/horitcultural/herding societies, the aged may still actively participate in the economic sphere—indeed, they may control it.

In stable agricultural societies, the aged also increasingly have come to control capital and property. By virtue of this economic control, the aged are able to achieve and to maintain high status in agricultural societies. A classic example of this can be seen in Ireland (27) where the high status of the elderly is closely tied to inheritance patterns. In

Ireland, fathers maintain control over the land until they are physically incapable of working it. Furthermore, before he is ready to retire, the father does not reveal which of his sons will be the recipient of the farm; thus, he is able to keep many sons around him as laborers. Fathers also do not typically allow their sons to marry until a very late age (perhaps in their 40s).

Moreover, with increased stability of residence, a food surplus can be built up, which can be shared with the aged in hard times. Surplus food also means that some members of society can be released from food-producing pursuits, and thus highly specialized professions in magic, curing, and politics can develop. Specialists in these areas can then barter reciprocally. Simmons (16) reports that among the Navajo, people bartered with old men for knowledge of magic songs, charms, and names, and that young men trained in magic were required to give their aged teachers large gifts, sometimes equal to half their earnings. In addition, certain old men could make a good living by performing healing rites.

Industrial Societies: In industrial societies the aged manage to exist and few are abandoned to the elements—although many are psychologically and geographically isolated. In these societies the aged are usually forced to leave gainful employment through compulsory retirement laws, even though they are not physically or mentally disabled. While the aged are usually provided with the minimum requirements for life through retirement pensions, they generally receive smaller proportions of wealth from the society than do the younger, economically productive members.

In capitalistic societies, the older person's control over the economic sphere decreases. The aged do not own or control the means of production because in most cases this is under the control of a corporate group, not the elder in a lineage or extended family. Hence, while shelter, food, and health care are usually provided for the aged, their status is obviously not as high as in a society in which they still control the major aspects of production.

An exception to the industrial pattern is Russia, where McKain (20) reports that the elderly are quite respected. One reason is that the elderly lead active and useful lives. Their pensions and fringe benefits enable them to live much as they did during their working years. Thus, they do not experience a decrease in income level, as do most older people in America. Grandparents often live with their children and grandchildren and are valued family members because of their economic contribution, for the pension of the elderly person is a welcome supplement to the household budget. In addition, Soviets are able to obtain better homes if they can claim more people in the household when they apply for an apartment. Furthermore, the older person performs essential household tasks such as cleaning and food shopping, thereby freeing the mother for work outside the home.

Mastery of critical knowledge is a technoeconomic correlate that influences the status and treatment of the aged in various societies. In preliterate societies with oral traditions, the aged are the repositories of ritual and technical knowledge. In speaking of the Semai, a group of people in which the aged have a semimonopoly on knowledge, Dentan (12) noted "wisdom consists largely of the lifelong accumulation of personal experience. The older a Semai is, the more he knows and the greater his expertise at dealing with his fellows. Such wisdom merits respect." In hunting/gathering and agrarian societies, technical knowledge remains relatively stable. However, in industrialized societies, the rapidity of technological change mitigates against the status of the aged; progress makes their technical skills and knowledge obsolete.

Kinship Systems. Kinship and household patterns are closely linked to the technoeconomic system, for example, small nuclear families are most common among highly industrialized people; in agrarian societies large extended families tend to live together in one household. However, these topics will be considered separately, because family patterns have a distinct influence on the status and treatment of the aged.

As Simmons noted:

Social relationships have provided the strongest securities to the individual especially in old age. With vitality declining, the aged person has had to rely more and more upon personal relations with others, and upon the reciprocal rights and obligations involved. . . . Throughout human history, the family has been the safest haven for the aged. Its ties have been the most intimate and longlasting, and on them the aged have relied for greatest security (16, p.17).

In societies (particularly rural or agricultural) where the extended type of family is the model form, the household may function as the economic, ritual, political, and social unit. In prerevolutionary China, the lineage (extended family) was responsible for the education, religion, marriage, and productive work of all its members. The extended family was also responsible for caring for its dependent members: the children, the infirm, and the elderly. The clan leadership was held by the eldest male member of the lineage. The elder remained economically, politically, and ritually active and exerted considerable control over all lineage affairs. In societies organized around extended families, the children reside in the parental home long after they achieve adulthood. However, as the society becomes more industrialized, the family typically breaks into nuclear-family household structures and frequently exhibits a neolocal residence pattern. In the extended-family household, where the aged person is the controller of the unit, even adult children may live in the parental home and consider the house to belong to the elder. While most aged in industrialized societies live apart from their children, those who do not tend to "come to live" with the children and thus are in a dependent position as the "house guest."

Highly industrialized societies are characterized by a large degree of geographic mobility with resulting physical isolation of the aged from the rest of his family. Bonds of kinship weaken, and the aged may no longer retain authority over the behavior and life-style of the rest of the family. When the elder person lives alone, he or she usually is no longer a viable part of the economic unit and ceases to function as a religious or political leader. The family is no longer the most secure force in the life of the aged; the state bureaucracy provides the monthly pension and pays for medical expenses. There are few remaining reciprocal role relations between the aged parent and his adult child. In addition, the growing tendency to segregate the aged into separate retirement communities further impoverishes the familial roles of the elderly.

Thus, household and kinship patterns, while closely tied to the type of economic system, are themselves important factors influencing the status and treatment of the aged in a society.

Political Systems. Like the dominant household type, the dominant political system is also frequently correlated with the economic mode. Most hunting/gathering societies have headmen as leaders; agricultural societies are commonly ruled by lineage elders or chiefs; and industrial societies most often have state political systems.

In preindustrial societies, political leaders often fill an ascribed or hereditary position. The usual prerequisite for obtaining this status is to be the eldest living male in the lineage or to be a member of an older age-grade. Because he possesses the greatest societal knowledge and controls the economic sphere, the elder is easily accorded political leadership.

Speaking of the Igbo in Nigeria, Shelton (13) noted that the elders are the primary political group in the society and control the lives and destinies of others. Elders are considered to be intermediaries between the ancestral forces and the rest of the lineage—hence they control fertility, mortality, crops, and fortunes.

As Simmons noted:

> . . . political, judicial and civil preferment has provided a major field for effective social participation of aged people, particularly those who already had attained position of prominence and responsibility in the prime of their lives. The title, and often the office, of chieftainship has tended to be lifelong. Councilmen and elders have also not infrequently fulfilled their function into very late old age. Old men, moreover, might serve long and well as lawmakers, judges, and administrators of justice. Finally, as leaders of secret societies and initiatory rites, the aged have quite generally received deference, for they have, more often than not, been the ones who have controlled the "rites of passage" from immaturity and subordination to adulthood, status and privilege (16, p.130).

Clark (32) presents an interesting perspective of elders as community leaders. As elders take over the judgmental and moralistic functions of the clan or village, they are performing what Freudians would call the collective superego functions. She speculates that a sound basis for this role in the psychology of individual maturation exists, and she supports her reasoning by citing Butler's claim to have found evidence in clinical materials that ego functions weaken in normal aging, and superego functions heighten in a compensatory way. She notes that in traditional societies, this transition is institutionalized.

Gender Difference.   The gender of the aged person also affects status and treatment. Generally, in hunting/gathering societies, old women and men are afforded relatively equal status. However, among farmers and herders, aged men usually hold a higher social position than aged women. Men seem to have the highest status in societies in which patrilocal residence, patrilineal descent, bride price, an organized priesthood, and ancestor worship are practiced (16).

On reaching old age, women in preindustrial societies often enjoy greater influence, freedom, and prestige. Among the Kapauku, an elderly woman is freed from food taboos and from her husband's scoldings and beatings. Younger people treat her particularly well because they believe a woman's soul is particularly dangerous after she dies if she has been abused (11).

In many societies women are considered dangerous during their fertile years and are restricted by special taboos. After menopause, however, they are often freed from these biases and restrictions. They may no longer have to endure such taboos as eating apart from men, living in seclusion, and speaking only to women or a designated male group.

In traditional China, marriage was patrilocal and descent was patrilineal; in most cases the woman went to live in the house of her husband's father. The woman of the house was the mother-in-law, and the daughter-in-law was the most subordinate person in the family. Sons received more obvious affection from mothers than from fathers, and sons maintained strong ties with mothers. Because parental relationships were more important than spouse relationships, a woman did not develop her own sphere of influence until her sons married and she became the head of the household (22).

Interestingly, in societies in which aged women have been respected, old men have rarely been without respect; but prestige for aged men has offered no assurance of the same status for women. If either sex has experienced a loss of respect in old age, it has more likely been women than men.

However, in an industrial society, elderly men may find forced retirement from work a devastating experience. Present-day elderly women typically have not worked outside the home; thus they may not experience the significant decrease in social status of their male counterparts, since their work roles do not change remarkably.

Ritual Leadership.   Cowgill found that religious leadership is more likely to be an important role of the aged in primitive societies than in modern societies. He saw this as one aspect of the tradition-maintenance and culture-transmission function of the aged in preliterate societies (33). As discussed previously in the section on belief systems, religious leadership by the aged has often been bolstered by various degrees of ancestor worship. Older people have known some of the ancestors personally, and they, who are about to die, will thus have more ready access to and influence on such ancestors. Among African Dahomeans it is reported that in old age both men and women are greatly respected, for with age comes considered judgment and, more importantly, with age comes a close affinity to the ancestral dead (16).

In speaking of the Pima Indians, Munsell noted that among the functions of the aged in a traditional society is the preservation of tradition (34). With modernization, there is a decrease in the ritual importance of the aged. They are no longer the "primary culture bearers": the culture is changing too rapidly for them to keep up. As Shelton noted among the Igbo of Nigeria, the spread of Christian missions and schools contributed directly to the decline in the powers of ancestors and gods, and, in turn, decreased the importance of the old people in Igbo society (13).

Summary of Status and Treatment of the Aged

There is extensive cross-cultural variation in the status and treatment of the aged. Societies can be arrayed along a continuum based on the amount of power and control held by the elderly. The basis of this power and control may lie in the culture's value systems, belief systems, or specific dimensions of social organization (economic, kinship, political, sex role, and religious systems). Again, it is necessary to observe the configurational pattern of these elements and not to hold one element as deterministic. Most important, however, is the realization that the configurational system present in the United States only represents one of a number of possible structures.

Simmons has well summarized the cultural variation in status and treatment of the aged:

In final summary, it can be stated explicitly that in primitive societies aged men and women have been generally regarded as repositories of knowledge and imparters of valuable information, as specialists in dealing with the uncertain aleatory element, and as mediators between their fellows and the fearful supernatural powers. These qualifications have operated to give them key positions in a wide range of social activities. They have been esteemed as experts in solving the problems of life. They have supervised and instructed in the arts and crafts; and have initiated hazardous and important undertakings, such as house-building, boat construction, the planting and harvesting of crops, and warfare. They have been in constant demand for treating diseases, exorcising spirits, working charms, controlling the weather, conjuring enemies, and predicting the future. They have been accredited officiators in the great events of life, such as childbirth, childnaming, initiations, weddings, funerals, and 'the laying of ghosts.' They have also functioned frequently as leaders at social gatherings and as directors of games, songs, dances, and festivals. In fact, hardly any of the great and critical occasions of life have not been presided over and supervised by some aged men or women. Truly, they have been the guardians of life's emergencies, the custodians of knowledge and the directors of ceremonies and pastimes. In possession of such great influence they have been the chief conservatiors of the status quo. Finally, after death, they have become supernatural agents themselves, still expert in the tried and tested wisdom of the aged, and very jealous of any young upstarts who might presume to challenge or change the ancient folkways (16, pp. 175–176).

CONTROVERSIES IN TRANSCULTURAL GERONTOLOGY

There are a number of controversial issues in the study of the aged in general and particularly in the study of transcultural aging. In large part, controversies have arisen when generalizations have been made on the basis of data gathered from mainstream American society without taking into account the range of life-styles, status, and treatment of the aged in other cultures.

Is the Status of the Aged Inversely Proportional to the Degree of Modernization Within the Society?

This hypothesis has been most strongly proposed by Cowgill and Holmes in *Aging and Modernization.* These authors collected ethnographic accounts of aging in a number of different cultures. In an attempt to derive generalizations about behaviors that appear to be universal, they link the status of the aged with an independent variable identified as "the degree of modernization." The specific factors that they include in this measure of modernization are level of technology, degree of urbanization, rate of social change, and degree of westernization (4).

Their major hypothesis is that the roles and status of the aged vary systematically with the degree of modernization of society, and that modernization tends to decrease the relative status of the aged and to undermine their security within the social system.

However, in their choice of societies, they did not use standard sampling techniques. While the ethnographic data in their compiled articles are excellent, the sample size is not sufficiently large to warrant their generalizations. In addition, other elements contributing to status and treatment, such as value orientations and belief systems, were ignored.

Both Palmore (15) and Clark and Anderson (6) found exceptions to the pattern cited by Cowgill and Holmes. Clark and Anderson noted that in many less modern societies, as well as in Western ones, aging is accompanied by a loss of social prestige. They cited the Cree Indians of northern Canada as an example. As a hunting and gathering group, the Cree community values primarily a doing orientation; that is, men must strive for obvious achievement: social approval depends on strenuous activity.

Clark and Anderson further noted that just as primitive societies differ in the status accorded the aged, so too do more technologically advanced and literate peoples vary. In contrast to our own society is the status of the elderly in Korea. There, to reach the age of 60 puts one practically in the category of the immortals and constitutes one of the greatest possible events in a person's life. Clark and Anderson concluded that just as simpler tribal or folk societies do not always provide old age with significant functions, the more complex cultures do not invariably fail to do so.

Thus, while the degree of modernization is a significant parameter in the status and treatment of the elderly, it is not necessarily a deterministic factor.

Is Disengagement a Cultural Universal?

The theory of disengagement was developed by Cumming and Henry on the basis of a study of using healthy middleclass whites in Kansas City. The major features of the disengagement theory are that because of physical decline, the aged person must decrease his activities and relinquish his social roles; and furthermore, that both the aged person and society benefit from his withdrawal from society and increased preoccupation with himself. Cummings and Henry and their proponents such as Richik, Chuculate, and Kilnert (35) hold that this disengagement theory has cross-cultural validity, and that the disengagement of the elderly is a transcultural universal.

A number of investigators, however, have found evidence to contradict the disengagement theory. In looking at the activity levels of the aged in a number of societies, Cowgill and Holmes found that there is little semblance of disengagement in traditional Africa or Samoa, and whatever disengagement there is, is balanced by the re-engagement of old people into the roles of elders (4). They also noted that some disengagement occurs in Thailand, but the process is quite gradual and seldom complete. Similarly, older people in Mexico reduce their strenuous physical activity but usually remain fully involved in familial roles.

Others, too, have found the disengagement theory to be less than valid. Shelton notes that dependency and psychosenility tend to be rare among the Igbo and that if any disengagement occurs it may be seen rather with the nonengagement of the very young in Igbo society. (19). He concluded that senility and disengagement are rare because of the increased involvement of the elders in the most prestigious affairs of the community and the diminution of stressful situations as a person ages.

Shanas (10) also found equivocal results from a cross-cultural study of disengagement. Looking at data from both Poland and the United States, she found that while with advancing age old people apparently do become increasingly self-preoccupied, there is no evidence for the decrease in normative controls that is postulated in the disengagement theory. Shanas claims that her findings dispute the disengagement theory.

Kooy and van't Kooster-van Wingerden (36) also dispute the cross-cultural validity of the disengagement theory after studying the aged in an urban Netherland community. They found that while total role activity did decrease with advancing age, the higher the activity among the aged in their sample. They argued this could not be understood from a disengagement framework.

Finally, Gutman (25) studied the highland Druze in Galilee, Syria, and Israel. In this sample, he found that disengagement need not be compulsory, and that passivity is not inextricably tied to disengagement. On the contrary, the so-called passivity of older men can be the central and necessary component of his engagement with age-appropriate social roles, traditions, and associated normative controls.

Hence, from a variety of investigations we conclude that disengagement is not necessarily a cultural universal and, in fact, may not even be an appropriate explanation for the activity pattern of the aged in Western societies.

Do the Aged Comprise a Subculture in the United States?

An issue that commonly arises in transcultural nursing is which groups of people can be considered to constitute subcultures? Not infrequently, there is a tendency to see subcultural groups if not everywhere, at least in more places than they rightly belong. Simply because a class of people share some common characteristics does not mean that they necessarily also share a culture. Culture is a specific concept that includes shared beliefs, norms, values, and patterns of behavior that are learned through the socialization process. Each person brings to old age a culture derived particularly from the ethnic group in which he received his socialization. Subcultural values, beliefs, and norms of behavior are integrated into the person's personality during his early formative years.

Rose (37) and, more recently, Sullivan (38) have promoted the idea that the elderly in the United States constitute a subcultural group. This is an inappropriate designation of the term *subcultural group* for two reasons: First, the aged are typically the most traditionally based culture bearers (i.e., they are usually last to become acculturated to dominant American values and beliefs). Hence, minority elderly will tend to be more heterogenous than minority members of any other age group. Second, patterns of life that may *seem* to indicate homogeneity among mainstream elderly are not patterns that are selected but that are largely dictated (e.g., mandatory retirement laws and declining physical integrity). Furthermore, Rosow (39) has demonstrated that the elderly do not obtain a set of beliefs as a result of aging that differ from those of the young.

Most of what we think we know about the aged members of minority groups in America is based on myths or subculture stereotypes. Partly because the ethnic aged have only recently become an intense area of research, there is a dearth of reliable, in-depth studies of the aged of American minority groups. Furthermore, results of reported investigations have been equivocal; opposing investigators have studied the same ethnic groups (sometimes in divergent settings) and have reported vastly different data or interpretations and conclusions.

From literature and popular belief, it is often anticipated that ethnic elderly will automatically have warm, close family relationships. However, a number of studies have demonstrated that this is, at best, an idealistic version of ethnic life. As Simos (40) found with Jewish aged on the West Coast, family relationships are a function of many variables. Socioeconomic class does influence the life-style patterns of an ethnic group, and factors related to adaptations to poverty must be separated from ethnic subcultural patterns.

It is important to remember that ethnic elderly are not one group. The following groups have been found to experience aging differently, both from the dominant middle-class perspective, as well as from each other: Blacks (41–46), Ladinos (24, 47–50), Oriental-Americans (51–53). In addition, these groups are not, in themselves, homogeneous, and several variant subcultural configurations may be found within each. Hence, each ethnic group and its subdivisions must be examined separately.

As demonstrated previously in the comparison of the Ladino and Anglo value system, ethnic diversity may result in widespread differences in the status and treatment of the elderly. Because America is composed of groups of people with quite diverse ethnic origins, we find that the American elderly do not constitute a homogeneous subcultural group, but, in fact, demonstrate considerable heterogeneity.

IMPLICATIONS OF
THE CULTURAL PERSPECTIVE
FOR GERONTOLOGICAL NURSING

As seen in this chapter, aging is a social as well as a biological process. In making a holistic assessment of the elderly, health professionals must not neglect the cultural dimension. While a cardinal principle in transcultural health care is that the people must not be stereotyped on the basis of their subcultural affiliation, the cross-cultural perspective connotes several health care implications that can serve as *assessment cues.*

First, there may be a discrepancy in categorizing people as aged depending on which criteria are used by the subcultural group. As discussed, Maricopa Indians may consider themselves to be aged when they are in their fourth decade; conversely, Greek-Americans may consider themselves to be middle-aged when they are in their eighth decade. Consequently, health care professionals should not *assign* people to an age group merely on the basis of their chronological age but must assess the meaning of the age grouping for the client.

Second, the social status we ascribe to an aged person may not be congruent with the status assigned by his subcultural group. An aged Japanese client may expect a young nurse to treat him with great deference, and he may be shocked if she acts toward him in a casual or familiar manner.

Third, the value system of the subcultural group may powerfully influence health care planning with the client. With a strong collateral value orientation, working-class black families are more likely than middleclass white families to wish to keep infirm aged family members in the home. Nursing-home placement is usually a last choice in extended care options (55). In addition, belief systems of subcultural group members may vary considerably from those of the health professional. Variant religious beliefs, particularly those surrounding death, require extremely careful assessment.

Fourth, while health care professionals must be culturally sensitive to the ethnic diversity of all age groups, they must be particularly cognizant of life-style differences among the elderly. The ethnic aged are likely to be the most tenaciously traditional and least acculturated members of their subcultural group. More than other age groups, the elderly tend to maintain traditional (ethnic) dietary habits. They are also more likely to maintain traditional ideas about disease causation and folk therapy than other age groups. In addition, their communication patterns (particularly if their native language is not English) tend to vary more dramatically than those of other age groups from that of the health professional. Hence, while dietary patterns, folk medicine, and communication differences are essential assessment factors in working with any subcultural client, they are particularly important in planning care with the ethnic *aged*.

SUMMARY

From this rather cursory view of transcultural aging, the following points may be concluded:

1. Cultures differ both in age classifications systems and in the criteria used for determining when a person reaches the category of "old".
2. The status and treatment accorded to the aged varies in each society. A number of factors influence the way in which the aged are perceived and treated in any given society; these factors include the value and belief systems, social structural components (including economic, kinship, political, and religious configurations), and suprasystem variables (ecology and rate of culture change).
3. The status of the aged is related to, but not necessarily determined by, the degree of modernization within the society.
4. Disengagement is not a cross-cultural universal.
5. At least in the United States, the aged do not comprise their own subculture; in fact, they exhibit greater heterogeneity than do younger age groups.
6. The pattern of aging exhibited by dominant mainstream America represents only one of a number of possible configurations.
7. Holistic assessment of the older person requires careful consideration of cultural factors.

REFERENCES

1. Fuller C: Aging Among Southern African Bantu, in Cowgill D, Holmes L (eds.): *Aging and Modernization.* New York, Appleton-Century-Crofts, 1972, pp 51–72.
2. Leaf A: Getting old, in Katz S (ed): *Biological Anthropology*, San Francisco, WH Freeman, 1979, pp 291–299.
3. Novosti Press Agency: *Very old people in the USSR. Gerontologist* 10: 151–152, 1970.

4. Cowgill D, Holmes L: Summary and conclusions: the theory in review, in Cowgill D, Holmes L (eds): *Aging and Modernization,* New York, Appleton-Century-Crofts, 1972, pp 305–324.

5. Hamer J: Aging in a gerontocratic society: the Sidamo of southwest Ethiopia, in Cowgill D, Holmes L (eds): *Aging and Modernization,* New York, Appleton-Century-Crofts, 1972, pp 15–30.

6. Clark M and Anderson B: *Culture and Aging: An Anthropological Study of Older Americans.* Springifled, Ill, Charles C Thomas Publisher, 1967.

7. Mead M: Ethnological aspects of aging. *Psychosomatics* 8:33–37, 1967.

8. Holmes L: The role and status of the aged in a changing Samoa, in Cowgill D, Holmes L (eds): *Aging and Modernization,* New York, Appleton-Century-Crofts, 1972, pp 73–90.

9. Cowgill D: The role and status of the aged in Thailand, in Cowgill D, Holmes L (eds): *Aging and Modernization.* New York, Appleton-Century-Crofts, 1972, pp 91–102.

10. Shanas E: Aging and life space in Poland and the United States. *J Hlth Soc Behav* 11:182–190, 1970.

11. Pospisil L: *Kapuku Papuans and Their Laws.* Yale University Publications in Anthropology No. 54. New Haven, Conn, Yale University Press, 1958.

12. Dentan R: *The Samai: A Nonviolent People of Malaya.* New York, Holt, Rinehart and Winston, 1968.

13. Shelton A: The Aged and Eldership among the Igbo, in Cowgill D, Holmes L (eds): *Aging and Modernization.* New York, Appleton-Century-Crofts, 1972, pp 31–50.

14. Oliver D: *A Soloman Island Society.* Boston, Beacon Press, 1955.

15. Palmore E: Sociological aspects of aging, in Busse E, Pfeiffer E (eds): *Behavior and Adaptation in Late Life.* Boston, Little, Brown & Co 1969, pp 33–70.

16. Simmons L: *The Role of the Aged in Primitive Society.* New Haven, Conn Yale University Press, 1945.

17. King S: *Perceptions of Illness and Medical Practice.* New York, Russell Sage Foundation, 1962.

18. Kluckhohn F, and Strodbeck F: *Variations in Value Orientations.* New York, Row Peterson and Company, 1961, p 4.

19. Shelton A: Igbo Childrearing, Eldership and Dependence: A Comparison of Two Cultures. *Occasional Papers in Gerontology* 8:97–106, 1969.

20. McKain W: The aged in the USSR, in Cowgill D, Holmes L (eds): *Aging and Modernization.* New York, Appleton-Century-Crofts, 1972, pp 151–166.

21. Feder S: Aging in the kibbutz in Israel, in Cowgill D, Holmes L (eds): *Aging and Modernization.* New York, Appleton-Century-Crofts, 1972, pp 211–226.

22. Yang M: *A Chinese Village.* New York, Columbia University Press, 1945.

23. Hsu F: *Under the Ancestor's Shadow.* New York, Columbia University Press, 1948.

24. Clark M and Mendelson M: Mexican-American aged in San Francisco, in Sze W (ed): *Human Life Cycle*. 1979, pp 651–660.
25. Gutman D: Alternatives to disengagement: the old men of the highland Druze, in Levine R (ed): *Culture and Personality*. Chicago, Aldine, 1974, pp 232–245.
26. Plath D: Japan: The years after, in Cowgill D, Holmes L (eds): *Aging and Modernization*. New York, Appleton-Century-Crofts, 1972, pp 133–150.
27. Streib G: Old age in Ireland: demographic and sociological aspects, in Cowgill D, Holmes L (eds): *Aging and Modernization*. New York, Appleton-Century-Crofts, 1972, pp 167–182.
28. Mauss M: *The Gift*. New York, Norton, 1925.
29. Watanabe H: Subsistence and ecology of northern food gatherers, in Lee R, Devore I (eds): *Man the Hunter*. Chicago, Aldine, 1968, pp 69–77.
30. Turnbull C: *The Forest People*. New York, Simon and Schuster, 1961.
31. Lee R: What hunters do for a living, or how to make out on scarce resources, in Lee R, Devore I (eds): *Man the Hunter*. Chicago, Aldine, 1968, pp 30–48.
32. Clark M: Cultural values and dependency in later life. *Occasional Papers in Gerontology* 8:59–72, 1969.
33. Cowgill D: A theory of aging in cross-cultural perspective, in Cowgill D, Holmes L (eds): *Aging and Modernization*. New York, Appleton-Century-Crofts, 1972, pp 1–14.
34. Munsell M: Functions of the aged among salt river pima, in Cowgill D, Holmes L (eds): *Aging and Modernization*. New York, Appleton-Century-Crofts, 1972, pp 127–132.
35. Richek H, Chuculate O, Klinert D: Aging and ethnicity in healthy elderly women. *Geriatrics* 26:146–152, 1971.
36. Kooy G, van't Klooster-van Wingerden C: The aged in an urban community in the Netherlands. *Human Development* 11:64–77, 1968.
37. Rose A: The subculture of the aging, in Rose A, Peterson W (eds): *Older People and Their Social World*. Philadelphia, FA Davis, 1965, pp 3–16.
38. Sullivan T: Some values, beliefs, and practices of the elderly in the United States: implications for health and nursing care. *Transcultural Nursing Care* 2:13–26, 1977.
39. Rosow I: *Social Integration of the Aged*. New York, Free Press, 1967.
40. Simos B: Relations of adults with aging parents. *Gerontologist* 10:135–139, 1970.
41. Moore J: Situational factors affecting minority aging. *Gerontologist* 11(suppl):88–93, 1971.
42. Jackson, JJ: Social gerontology and the Negro: a review. *Gerontologist* 7:168–178, 1967.
43. Jackson JJ: Aged Negroes: their cultural departures from statistical stereotypes and rural-urban differences. *Gerontologist* 10:140–145, 1970.
44. Jackson JJ: Negro aged: toward needed research in social gerontology. *Gerontologist* 11(suppl):52–57, 1971.
45. McCaslin R, Calvert W: Social indicators in black and white: some ethnic

considerations in delivery of services to the elderly, *J Gerontol* 30:60–66, 1975.
46. Jackson, JS, Bacon J, Peterson J: Life satisfaction among black urban elderly, *J Aging Human Development.* 8:169–179, 1977.
47. Carp F: Communicating with elderly Mexican-Americans. *Gerontologist* 10:126–133, 1970.
48. Clark M: *Health in the Mexican-American Culture* Berkeley, University of California Press, 1970.
49. Moore J: Mexican-Americans. *Gerontologist* 11 (suppl):30–35, 1971.
50. Maldonado D: The Chicano Aged. *Social Work* 20:213–216, 1975.
51. Kalish R, Yuen S: Americans of East Asian ancestry: aging and the aged. *Gerontologist* 11(suppl):36–47, 1971.
52. Carp F, Kataoka E: Health care problems of the elderly of San Francisco's Chinatown. *Gerontologist* 16:30–38, 1976.
53. Roberts W: All in the family: the older person in context; in Bauwens E (ed): *The Anthropology of Health*. St. Louis, CV Mosby, 1978, pp 177–191.
54. Nobles W, Nobles G: African roots in black families: the social-psychological dynamics of black family life and the implications for nursing care, in Luckraft D (ed): *Black Awareness: Implications for Black Patient Care.* New York, American Journal of Nursing Company. 1976, pp 6–11.

ANNOTATED BIBLIOGRAPHY

Cowgill D, Holmes L (eds): *Aging and Modernization.* New York, Appleton-Century-Crofts, 1972.
A collection of 19 articles primarily dealing with the experience of aging in nonAmerican settings. Ethnographic articles represent a variety of tribal as well as industrial societies. Theoretical articles deal with the effect of modernization on the status and treatment of the elderly.
Leininger M (ed): *Transcultural Nursing Care of the Elderly.* Salt Lake City, University of Utah, 1977.
A collection of eight articles focusing on American ethnic aged and implications of divergent life-styles for health care.
Simmons L: *The Role of the Aged in Primitive Society.* New Haven, Conn, Yale University Press, 1945.
Virtually the first and only comprehensive cross-cultural study of aging. Using data gathered from the Human Area Relations File, Simmons addresses the following topical areas: assurance of food; property rights; prestige, general activity, political and civil activities, use of knowledge, magic and religion, functions of the family, and reactions to death.

chapter three
physical health
in the second half
of life

Remember your Creator in the days of your youth,
before the days of trouble come and the years
    approach when you will say,
"I find no pleasure in them"
before the sun and the light and moon
    and the stars grow dark,
and the clouds return after the rain;
when the keepers of the house tremble,
    and the strong men stoop,
when the grinders cease because they are few,
and those looking through the windows grow dim;
    and when the doors to the street are closed
    and the sound of grinding fades;
when men rise up at the sound of birds, but all
    their songs grow faint;
when men are afraid of heights and of dangers
    in the streets;
when the almond tree blossoms and the grasshopper
    drags himself along and desire no longer is stirred.
Then man goes to his eternal home and mourners go
    about the streets.

Ecclesiastes 12: 1–5
The Holy Bible, *NIV*

OUTLINE

BIOLOGICAL THEORIES OF AGING: AN OVERVIEW
Introduction
Historical Approaches to Theories of Aging
Current Biological Theories of Aging
Conclusion
THE TRIAD OF REST, ACTIVITY, AND NUTRITION
Introduction
Adequate Rest
Physical Activity
Nutrition and The Elderly Client
Assessment of the Client's Use of Medication
MODIFYING PHYSICAL ASSESSMENT PARAMETERS TO
EVALUATE THE OLDER CLIENT
Introduction
The Integument
The Eye and Vision
The Ear and Hearing
The Nose and Oral Cavity
The Respiratory System
The Cardiovascular System
The Musculoskeletal System
The Neurological System
The Genitourinary System
SUMMARY

BIOLOGICAL THEORIES OF AGING: AN OVERVIEW

Introduction

It is an accepted fact that biological aging occurs in all living organisms. Biological aging is a natural process that is initiated at conception and is under the direction of a person's genetic makeup. Aging in the human species is often defined in terms of physical changes, which are observed both by the person who is aging and by those with whom he or she interacts. Of these observations, skeletal and integumentary changes are usually the most obvious. However, these changes are often so gradual that the person who is advancing in years chronologically, and who thinks of himself as healthy, hardly notices them.

Reference to the physical changes of aging is usually made in terms of the concept of loss. Indeed, much of what actually occurs with biochemical or physiological aging is either a loss or decrease of a molecular, cellular, tissue, or organ function. Since the terms *loss* and *decrease* are usually perceived as negative, biological aging is frequently viewed as an overwhelmingly negative experience. Such negative viewpoints can have a major influence on the psychosocial components of aging for individuals and groups.

Historical Approaches to Theories of Aging

The observation that humans have always been interested in the aging process was made in Chapter 1; however, this interest was often focused on finding ways to prevent aging. For example, ancient Egyptians sought the elixir that would provide eternal youth; and in the thirteenth century, Roger Bacon saw aging as a disease process that could be stopped by good hygiene.

Throughout history, others dealt with the reality of physical aging by emphasizing the philosophical components of life. The ancient Chinese saw aging as a good thing in that long life symbolized that a person had lived a good life. The Hindu belief in reincarnation is an approach to aging that focuses on the metaphysical rather than the biological processes.

Biological aging as described by the "teacher" in Ecclesiastes, although in poetic terms, refers to generalized deterioration and eventual physical death.

Hippocrates (460–377 BC) was the first person in recorded history to theorize about aging. He saw aging as a natural and irreversible phenomenon that resulted from a decrease in body heat. Galen (130–201 AD) proposed a similar theory and said that the increased dryness and coldness of aging were a function of changes in body humors.

Leonardo da Vinci's (1452–1519) clear descriptions and drawings of anatomical findings, during autopsies in people of all ages, facilitated later development of theories of biological aging. From the seventeenth through the nineteenth centuries theories with various emphases developed, such as hardening of body fibers, loss of tissue irritability, and a change in the vital force or spirit.

Despite this long history of interest in the aging process, systematic research on the process of biological aging is a recent development. Much research has taken place since the early 1950s, both in Europe and the United States. Aging research, gerontology, and geriatric medicine are phenomena of the twentieth century.

Current Biological Theories of Aging

The task of outlining current, prevailing theories of biological aging succinctly is unquestionably a formidable one. Scientists have approached the aging process from their own professional perspectives rather than in an interdisciplinary manner. Therefore, there are genetic, chemical, pathological, and morphological explanations of the aging process. Possibly the only area of agreement in aging research is that there is very little likelihood of ever identifying one unifying theory of biological aging. However, some concept of genetic instability comes closest to a unifying theory of aging, and genetic concepts are involved in most theories of aging.

It seems appropriate to differentiate between theories of aging and certain processes that take place within the aging organism in spite of the necessary overlap between these two categories. For a clear discussion of biological aging, it is necessary first to examine some of the commonly occurring aging processes, for these processes are frequently the bases for the various theories of aging.

A significant finding of aging research is that there is a limit to the number of times cells replicate themselves. In 1961 Hayflick and Moorhead reported their findings that there are limits to the number of times normal diploid human fibroblasts can replicate themselves in vitro. Since that time, these findings have been confirmed by other researchers. Hayflick reports that "the sum of population doublings undergone by normal fetal human fibroblasts both before and after preservation is always equal to 50 ± 10" (1). Moreover, cells isolated from older people undergo progressively fewer doublings before stopping (2). As a result of these studies the cultured human fibroblast has become a widely used object of research into the fundamental cause(s) of aging.

Other researchers have found that as an organism ages the functional capacity of the homeostatic mechanisms that govern immunity decreases. It has also been observed that as organisms age, both the cell division process and RNA synthesis slow down. In addition, as an organism ages, there is an increasing heterogeneity of cells, that is, cells vary more in size, shape, and in mitotic capabilities. Cristofalo (3) found an "increase in lysosomal enzyme activity" both in biochemical and ultrastructure studies. It has been suggested that lysosomes degenerate and that in some tissues lipofuscin, the "aging pigment," derives from such lysosomes.

Possibly the most encompassing observation is that of the phenomenon of increasing collagen cross-linking with aging, which was made in the early 1950s by Fritz Verzar and other researchers in Switzerland. Other studies have confirmed this observation and stimulated additional research on this phenomenon. Kohn, who has written extensively on his work in this area, believes that, in examining research findings, mechanisms that require few assumptions should be more readily accepted than those that require many assumptions. In this connection he says, "we might assume that the major manifestations of age result from one change or a small number of changes in a system that is common to all organs" (4). He proceeds to describe "a progressive intermolecular cross-linking of collagen" as the "most characteristic age change" that can be observed in many body parts.

According to Kohn, collagen:

> . . . constitutes 25 to 30 percent of the total body protein [and] is distributed in and around walls of all blood vessels and around cells. . . . It functions to maintain form and to limit deformation of tissues. . . . Progressive cross-linking of collagen, which appears to occur throughout the body, would tend to interfere with the flexibility of fibrils and thereby make tissues less mobile. . . . Since all physiological processes depend on tissue movement and diffusion of substances, the generalized physiological decline with age could be explained on these bases. An impaired passage of gases, nutrients, metabolites, hormones, antibodies, and accumulated toxins would, furthermore, explain why aging animals become increasingly susceptible to being killed by miscellaneous diseases, injuries, and insults. Some cell death and altered function secondary to altered passage of materials would be expected (4, pp.209–210, 213).

In many ways the collagen cross-linking that takes place as an animal ages seems to be very significant in theory development. "The view that macromolecular cross-linking causes aging is a variation of one of the oldest theories of aging—that aging is caused by syneresis of body colloids" (4). Thus, "when Leonardo da Vinci claimed that aging was due to thickening of tunics of veins that restricted the passage of blood, he may not have been very far from the truth" (4).

One approach to outlining theories of senescence or biological aging is to divide them into two categories: those based on active processes, and those based on passive processes. Passive process theories refer to the process of wearing out, which has variously been called tissue wear and tear, an accumulation of inert or harmful substances, a progressive asynchrony of activities, an accumulation of errors, or a gradual accumulation of irreparable damage. For example, random genetic changes could be classified as a passive aging process . Also, it has been shown that the body loses the ability to retain the "optical purity" of biomolecules, as demonstrated by the fact that not all of the amino acids have the L-configuration. This, too, may be a passive process of aging (5).

Active process theories point to age-dependent deterioration as the result of an active "self-destruct" program. The most supportable of these theories is that based on the broad concept of genetic programming. However, there is much disagreement on what form genetic programming or genetic instability takes.

Currently, genetic theories assume that aging is specified by the DNA in each species. The specific hypotheses are that alterations of the DNA code, or of the transcription or translation of that code, are the causes of aging. One theory, which has lost some of its former support, is that of somatic mutation. This theory states that there is an increased frequency of chromosomal aberrations within cells during aging. However, there has been a fair amount of research that does not support this theory.

Chemical research into the presence and changes in free radical formation relates in some ways to genetic theories. Free radicals may bind with DNA and thus alter its configuration, causing cellular mutation. Although the free radical theory of aging is not widely supported, none of the evidence found has been refuted nor is the theory easily explained (5). It is known that the bombardment of cells by x-ray beams can cause ionization of free radicals. The free radical theory may also relate to the autoimmune theories of aging (6).

Autoimmune theories have a somewhat tenuous basis in current research. These theories are based on the observations that aging is "accompanied by decreased functional capacity of the homeostatic mechanism governing immunity" (7), and that there is an increased percentage of abnormal serum globulins and autoantibodies in aging populations. The presence of increased autoantibodies and decreased homeostatic capacity may cause tissue damage and may increase susceptability to some infectious processes. However, to say that autoimmunity is a cause of aging is not supported by present research data.

There are a few persons who would describe biological aging as a disease process. In doing this, they refer to aging as being caused by either a latent or slow virus infection. However, there is little evidence to support such an hypothesis.

As was mentioned earlier, it does seem that the collagen cross-linkage theory is more complete and unifying than many other theories. However, fundamental questions still remain: What is the cause of the process of collagen cross-linkage? Does it occur in response to a genetic program that was established at conception for the specific organism? Does it relate to the amount of biochemical stress with which the organism has had to cope?

It has been observed by Kohn and others that while an organism is growing, the cross-linkage process is slow or nonexistent. However, when maturity has been achieved, cross-linkage of collagen occurs more rapidly. Does this then, bring us back to the genetic program idea? Is the plan for aging passed from generation to generation? Can biological aging be described as the ultimate result of the growth and development process?

Conclusion

Regardless of whether or not the exact causes of aging can be isolated, many biophysiological and biochemical changes, which occur as an organism ages, have been identified. Some of these changes are harmful, that is, they interfere with the efficient, healthy function of cells, tissues, organs, and organisms. Other changes are seen as incidental with no apparent detrimental effects.

Research into the process of aging continues to be of importance; however, the likelihood of preventing the process and its ultimate end, death, is minuscule. Of greater importance is the identification of causes and characteristics of the harmful effects of aging so these effects can be delayed or decreased. The value of such findings would be in the improvement of the quality of life while the quantity of life is increased.

THE TRIAD OF REST, ACTIVITY, AND NUTRITION

Introduction

Support continues to increase for the notion that certain health practices tend to inhibit biological aging and promote physical health. Health behaviors thus identified are appropriately advocated by the professional nurse since promotion of health and prevention of illness are among nursing's primary goals. However, care must be taken at this juncture not to equate biological aging with illness.

When the nurse assesses the health status of an elderly client, collecting data about certain health practices is important. In addition, a client's description of what he or she believes to be good health practice provides essential clues during a holistic assessment process.

Health practices and health behaviors have been variously defined and studied in medical, public health, nursing, and behavioral science literature. Definitions of *health* range from "the mere absence of illness" to a "dynamic state of well being." Dunn defines the latter as "high level wellness," which he describes as "an integrated method of functioning which is oriented toward maximizing the potential of which the individual is capable" (8).

Researchers in Finland defined health behavior as "any activity undertaken by a person believing himself to be healthy, for the purpose of preventing disease or detecting it in an asymptomatic stage." They found that persons who believed themselves to be healthy did not consider diet to be of much importance; however, there was significantly "less illness among those with an active interest in physical exercise and with a restrictive attitude to smoking and drinking" (9).

Belloc and Breslow (10) looked at the relationship of health status to health practices in 6,928 adult subjects who were followed for over five years. They found that life expectancy and improved health are related in a significant way to eating regular meals three times a day as opposed to snacking, eating breakfast every day, exercising moderately, getting seven to eight hours of sleep, maintaining moderate weight, not smoking, and not drinking alcoholic beverages or drinking moderately. These data provide evidence that health practices do influence health status.

Adequate rest, regular physical activity, and proper nutrition are the three health practices emphasized most frequently in the literature. Moreover, these behaviors are interdependent. For example, the person who has a regular routine of physical activity burns up more calories than a sedentary person. In addition, physical activity tends to increase circulation and to promote relaxation, thereby improving sleep. An example of this interdependence comes to us from history. Thomas Jefferson "attributed the hardiness of his constitution to a regimen of daily riding, bathing the feet in ice-water, and drinking and eating sparingly, particularly of meat" (11). Too many people, of all ages, have lulled themselves into a comfortable, but deadly, life-style that includes little or sporadic exercise, relaxation by participating in sedentary activities, and stuffing themselves with high caloric snacks which are often low in food value.

Adequate Rest

Adequate rest was operationally defined by Belloc and Breslow as seven to eight hours of sleep during a 24-hour period. However, individual variations from this norm need to be taken into account when assessing a person's rest or sleep status. In addition, rest is more important than sleep, although sleep "appears to be the primary and most imperative form of rest" (12). Other components of the concept of rest include relaxation, leisure activities, and diversion from the normal routine. These components, somewhat elusive and not well-defined in the literature, overlap some with physical activity.

Research into sleep patterns has established that sleep is a cyclical component of an organism's circadian rhythm. Not only is sleep correlated with the low temperature portion of a person's 24-hour temperature rhythm but also sleep has its own predictable rhythmicity. Experiments that measure brain activity and muscle movement, along with vital signs information, have revealed the pattern of sleep stages during a night of sleep (13).

Sleep can be divided into two general categories: the slow wave sleep periods and the rapid eye movement (REM) sleep periods. Slow wave sleep periods are further divided into four stages, differentiated by electrophysiological techniques. The characteristics of the various periods and stages of sleep are outlined on Table 5.

When assessing sleep and rest in an older population, the normal variations in sleep patterns that occur with the aging process need to be considered. During the past two decades, studies have demonstrated that as a person reaches adulthood, slow wave sleep periods decrease. For example, in the first sleep cycle of a given night, the slow wave sleep period for a young child may be 100 to 120 minutes. However, by the time a person reaches the mid-teen years, the slow wave sleep period in the first cycle of sleep is usually only about 60 minutes and remains relatively stable throughout the remainder of life.

However, studies have shown that, as a person enters the middle years, the slow wave sleep periods lengthen somewhat throughout the sleep cycles of a given episode of sleep. At the same time, the length of the rapid eye movement (REM) sleeping period decreases during the sleep cycles as the person ages (see Fig. 5).

The other finding of interest is that the awakenings that take place during a period of sleep last longer for the older person; that is, the person in his or her 20s, when aroused or awakened typically will stay awake for two to five minutes, irrespective of the sleep cycle in which

Table 5. Characteristics of Sleep Periods and Stages

Periods	Muscle Action	EEG Patterns	Vital Signs	Subjective Awareness
Slow Wave Sleep				
Stage 1	Relaxing	Low amplitude	Respirations more even, pulse slower	Floating sensation, "borderline" consciousness, may be dreaming
Stage 2	Relaxed	Low amplitude, fast frequency		Sleeping soundly, easily awakened
Stage 3	Very relaxed	High amplitude, slow frequency 20 to 50% of time	Respirations even, pulse slows more, temperature drops	Fairly loud noise required to awaken
Stage 4	Very relaxed movement rare	Same as stage 3 but 50% of time		Oblivious sleep, difficult to awaken; when awakened, focuses slowly
REM sleep	Increased activity	Same as stage 2, accompanied by rapid eye movement	Pulse rises, respirations more rapid, BP rises	Vivid dreaming, hard to awaken

the arousal occurs. On the other hand, the person who is in his or her seventies may stay awake 5 to 20 minutes, depending on the sleep cycle in which the arousal takes place (see Fig. 5).

There is very little agreement among the sleep researchers about the significance of these variations, and there is little agreement on the value of REM sleep. Different people hypothesize different purposes; some say the REM sleep period has little effect on sleep quality. If this is so, what is the reason then for REM rebound? REM rebound is the response that follows a period of REM sleep deprivation in which there is a great increase in the amount of REM sleep on nights immediately following REM sleep deprivation (15). This phenomenon has not been conclusively associated with any specific illness or health problem. For example, Feinberg found that even when REM sleep was entirely suppressed, there was no obvious detriment to humans (16). He concludes that, whereas REM sleep could be dispensed with, slow wave sleep periods seemed essential to the health and well-being of humans.

It is interesting to note that the total number of minutes spent per night in the slow wave sleep period does increase as a person ages (see Fig. 5). The reason for this is unclear, but problems associated with lack of sleep seem to relate more closely to a decrease in slow wave sleep than to lessened REM sleep. One explanation relates to a person's developmental needs. For instance, an infant may need high levels of REM sleep to stimulate maturation of the sensory system.

Moreover, periods of waking increase with age. Possibly these periods of waking are necessary to compensate for the decrease in total REM sleep in the older person. On the other hand, the periods of waking for older people are often long enough that they are truly aware of being awake. This may be the reason why older people sometimes complain about not being able to sleep as well as when they were younger. Also the sleep of an older person seems not to be as deep as the sleep of a younger person in that stages 3 and 4 of the slow wave sleep period decrease in length or are nonexistent for the older person. Therefore, the older person is less likely to be "dead to the world" when asleep than the younger person.

The question then is—what is adequate sleep for an elderly person?

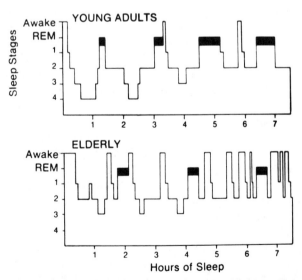

Figure 5. Sleep cycle changes with aging. (Reproduced with permission, Kales, Anthony, The UCLA interdepartmental conference, sleep and dreams. *The Annals of Internal Medicine,* Vol. 68:1081, 1968.)

Any definition of adequate rest or sleep needs to be perceived as a guideline and not as an absolute requirement. In addition to the individual variations and changes related to aging, it is important to remember that rest is only one component of a person's life-style and health behavior. Therefore, viewing the whole person is of utmost importance. What is the client's perception of his or her normal sleep experience? After the nurse has collected this information, data about the causes of the variations in the usual sleep and rest patterns should be collected. What physical, personal, environmental, or social factors make it difficult for the client to obtain what he or she perceives to be adequate rest? Does he or she believe that variations in sleep cause a feeling of not having rested upon arising? Do the responsibilities or roles of the client influence the quality of sleep or rest achieved? Moreover, what value does the client place on rest or sleep? Are rest or sleep seen as essential to good health, or would the client prefer to use the time spent resting in some other way?

Although a nurse's knowledge of research data and therapeutic guidelines is basic in a holistic assessment process, the client's perceptions of his or her health status are the most important data that can be collected during the assessment phase of the nursing process. A client may report an average of eight hours of sleep per night, but if he or she believes that is not personally healthy, a need exists that requires further assessment and subsequent intervention.

Furthermore, are rest and sleep used as ways of coping with decision making, boredom, or problems? For example, a person who has recently experienced a loss may spend more than his or her usual amount of time sleeping. Subjective tiredness or the desire to withdraw from experiencing the pain of a loss may be motives for increasing the time spent sleeping or resting. On the other hand, reminiscence and the desire to think about the object of a loss could cause a person to have difficulty sleeping or resting.

In addition, health teaching is an important component of the intervention phase of the nursing process. The nurse may find, after assessing a client's rest/sleep status, that some teaching about normal changes in sleep patterns is advisable. Knowledge that such changes are normal in healthy people as they age may alleviate the anxiety associated with experiencing these changes.

Earlier it was mentioned that rest is more important than sleep, and that certain activities are often perceived as restful. The topic of physical activity is tied very closely to the topic of rest. In fact, they are interrelated in that physical activity often provides the physiological stimulus for improved sleep.

Physical Activity

Americans have become progressively more sedentary during the twentieth century. This is partly true because jobs demand less physical activity, transportation is usually sedentary, and home care and maintenance are increasingly mechanized. Along with the sedentary work environment has come an increase in psychosocial and work-related tension and stress. "Such overstress and under-exercise causing 'hypokinetic disease' can accelerate premature aging. On the other hand, proper exercise contributes to longevity and preserves function in old age" (17). Although it is true that physical strength and flexibility normally decrease somewhat with aging, many studies and subjective, personal testimonies attest to this decrease being much more gradual when people remain physically active as a matter of routine.

In a retrospective study with 568 matched pairs of men, researchers found that "increased leisure activity, but not job-related physical activity, is associated with a lowered risk of coronary death." They concluded that "increased leisure activity can contribute to the prevention of death due to coronary heart disease" (19). These findings are consistent with prospective studies that show that regular activity facilitates good health even in an environment where sedentary jobs are common.

The focus of this book is on older people, but the ideal for physical activity, which results in improved physical health, is a life-long lifestyle of physical activity and fitness. However, it has been shown that even when people are in their middle or older years, initiation and consistent involvement in a program of gradually increasing physical exercise improves physical and mental fitness, vigor, and enjoyment of life for many people. It is important to point out at this juncture that a sedentary older person should have a complete physical examination before embarking on a program of physical exercise. Such an examination provides the information needed by the client's physican to provide specific recommendations about the amount and type of exercise the client engages in, at least initially. Even so, there is support in the literature for at least moderate exercise even for people with rather severe physical problems.

Physical activity usually improves health for people of all ages with few or no health problems by increasing flexibility, strength, and cardiorespiratory endurance. The person who decides to become involved in a program of physical exercise is advised to move gradually from current activity to the desired active level. By using a gradual approach to increasing physical activity, people can eventually be involved in activity that may be perceived as being quite strenuous.

Walking is described by many authorities as the safest and best exercise. Walking, if it is to improve a person's physical health, needs to be brisk, and consistent rather than casual and sporadic. Swimming is also recommended, since the water can provide buoyancy for a person who is experiencing joint pain or stiffness. Some exercises may be recommended, however, caution should be taken in use of anaeorbic or isometric exercise, since there is a "decrease of anaeorbic power with age" and "cerebral ischemia in strenuous exericse is probably more pronounced in older people" (20). Furthermore:

> Isometric exercise would be undesirable because not only are high levels of muscle contraction attained, but they are also maintained without the relaxation pauses provided by rhythmic activity during which blood flow is unresisted. Thus, we may conclude that exercise programs for older people should maximize the rhythmic activity of large muscle masses and minimize 1) high activation levels of small muscle masses and 2) static (or isometric) contractions. The natural activities of walking, jogging, running and swimming seem to be best suited to this purpose. (21, p.51).

The foregoing information on physical activity and aging provides the nurse with some basis for establishing assessment guidelines to evaluate a client's involvement in physical activity. However, the client's perception of his or her physical activity and associated feelings of physical health or illness are equally important. The nurse uses his or her knowledge of the importance of regular, moderate physical activity to the promotion of physical and emotional well-being as a baseline for assessing the client's perception of his or her physical activity and status.

Has the client's physical activity remained fairly constant throughout life? Or, did he or she on retirement, cease being active? What does the client believe is good health practice in relation to physical activity? What is the client's evaluation of his or her present physical activity and status in comparison to a month ago, a year ago, five years ago, and so forth? How often has he or she consulted a health professional or some other source for guidance in relation to physical activity?

Although the primary focus of this book is the nurse's role in assessment of a client, the importance of the nursing profession's role in health education to promote health and general well-being should also be emphasized. The nurse has an important role, along with other health professionals to teach individuals and groups about the value of consistent, regular physical activity. Client education is important but should not precede a thorough health history and physical assessment to determine the client's knowledge, beliefs, and current health status.

Nutrition and the Elderly Client

Of the topics rest, activity, and nutrition, nutrition is discussed in the literature more often in relation to aging that are the others. Although nutrition seems to have high priority among health professionals who work with elderly clients, it is of less importance than rest and activity to many elderly persons who see themselves as healthy. Dietary habits, just as rest and activity patterns, are likely to remain much as they were for decades for the older person who has no nutritionally related health problems.

Although considerable research has been done to ascertain the age changes associated with nitrogen balance and protein synthesis, findings are equivocal (22). Such information could provide guidelines for the determination of minimum or recommended nutritional needs of the elderly. Continued investigation into the biochemical bases of nutritional needs of the elderly is an important area of research.

Generally speaking, from the information currently available, the nutrition requirements of older people are similar to those of adults of any age. The one difference usually mentioned in the literature is that total caloric requirements are less. Total calorie requirements decrease slightly as a person ages, because of cellular level changes and a lower basal metabolic rate. Decreased physical activity also decreases caloric needs (23).

Various guidelines are available to use in assessing the adequacy of a client's nutrient intake. However, the most useful of these is the Recommended Dietary Allowances (revised in 1974), which is outlined by the Food and Nutritional Board of the National Research Council (24), because the needs of different age groups are outlined. For example, the RDA for men and women over 51 years of age are as follows. A man who weighs 70 kg (154 pounds) has energy requirements of around 2,400 calories/day. A woman weighing 58 kg (128 pounds) needs about 1,800 calories/day to meet her energy needs. RDAs of vitamins and minerals for people over 51 years of age are similar to the RDAs for younger adults. This information refers, of course, to the person without nutritionally related illness.

Nutritional guidelines, just as any other guidelines, need to be perceived as average, and individual differences should be taken into consideration. The client who is fairly active, feels vigorous and healthy, and does not demonstrate any significant weight change is very likely receiving adequate nutrition. However, assessment of dietary habits and physical examination, with nutritional guidelines in mind, is essential in holistic assessment.

Studies have shown that a three-day record of a client's dietary intake provides an accurate assessment of eating habits (25). This record should be compared with one of the established nutritional guidelines to determine if there are any caloric, vitamin, or mineral deficiencies or excesses. If a client has a nutritionally associated health problem, appropriate adjustments would need to be made. For instance, an obese person who is on a diet should obviously have a lower caloric intake than the charts would show for a person of that age and weight. Vitamin and mineral needs, however, would remain constant for such a person.

Nutritionally related physical assessment includes observation for skin or hair dryness. Some skin lesions and capillary fragility may indicate vitamin deficiencies. Oral tenderness, redness, bleeding, or ulceration may indicate one or more vitamin deficiencies. Persons exhibiting these symptoms usually should be referred to a physician for a more complete evaluation.

Dietary studies of older people in the United States and Great Britain have revealed a few significant deficiency problems. Calcium and protein deficiencies were most common, but vitamin and caloric deficiencies were also found. A great problem was the excessive intake of calories, especially with the use of foods high in calories and low in nutrient value. Excessive intake of vitamins and minerals, often in the form of over-the-counter medication, was also found. However, obesity and high blood pressure are more likely nutritionally related problems for older people than are diseases that result from vitamin deficiencies (24–29).

A moderate number of older people, who see themselves as healthy, have chronic health problems that are at least partially controlled by special diets. For example, cardiac problems may require a low-salt diet. However, special diets will not be discussed here since they are not typical for a person who is physically healthy. This is not to say that special diets do not promote health, but rather that the focus and space in this book does not allow for an indepth review of special diets which may promote health for a minority of older clients. Nutrition textbooks provide indepth coverage of special diet information for the nurse.

Although nutrition is appropriately discussed in the physical health category of a holistic approach to clients, knowledge about good nutrition and attitudes about food are also important to nutritional behavior. In fact, various authors have listed ignorance of good nutrition, social isolation, and economic problems as primary causes of nutritional deficiencies.

In most cultures, eating is a social activity. When an older person has experienced the loss of a significant other with whom he or she lives, he or she may become less interested in eating for various reasons and may, therefore, change eating habits and develop nutritional problems (30).

Discovery of inadequate dietary intake during a complete health assessment also may provide clues about the person's financial needs. Personal pride and the need to remain self-sufficient sometimes prevents people from sharing such information. The nurse should be sensitive to the client's needs and right to privacy. She or he may provide information about resources commonly available in the client's community to alleviate economically related nutritional problems without learning the details of his or her financial status.

Assessment of Client's Use of Medication

Drugs and Nutrition

A frequently overlooked element in nutritional assessment is the effect of drugs on the body's use of nutrients. Drugs can cause gastrointestinal inflammation. They can interfere with enzyme activity, change the gastric pH, and bring about an electrolyte imbalance (31). These factors can result in changes in the absorption of nutrients, vitamins, and minerals.

People who are chronic users of antacids, whether under medical supervision or by self-prescription of over-the-counter (OTC) preparations, may develop thiamine deficiency, since part of the absorption process occurs in the duodenum. Antacids, such as Rolaids, that contain sodium may interfere with the efficacy of low-salt diets or may counteract the effectiveness of diuretic drugs.

The frequent use of cathartics may decrease nutrient absorption since the increased gastrointestinal activity may cause the digestive process to speed up and decrease the time during which absorption can occur. Indiscriminate use of cathartics can also cause fluid and electrolyte imbalance. This may occur more quickly in an elderly person since the body's ability to maintain electrolyte equilibrium decreases with aging.

Importance of Drug Use Assessment

Data on the client's use of medication are important to collect during the history-taking component of the nursing assessment. Drugs not only effect a person's gastrointestinal system but also have systemic and generalized effects that may extend beyond the purpose intended by a physician or by the client who chooses to practice self-prescription by using OTC remedies. Often a client's lack of knowledge about both the intended action of a drug and its potentially harmful side effects results in the simultaneous use of several medications that can have adverse effects. In addition, if a client sees several doctors for different health problems, the problems of mixing drugs in a potentially danger- ous manner may arise. In drug interaction, some drugs potentiate the action of others, sometimes to an overdose level. Other drugs inhibit the action of other drugs, sometimes completely neutralizing their ac- tion. The possibility of toxic results from drug combinations also exists.

An example of a potentially harmful drug combination is Valium (Diazepam), a commonly prescribed, fairly mild sedative-antianxiety drug, and alcohol. Since older people may consume moderate amounts of wine or "therapeutic toddies" or they may use OTC alcohol- containing cough remedies, and liquid vitamin supplements, clients using Valium need to be told about the dangers of mixing alcohol and Valium. This is only one of many examples of drug interactions that can be harmful when the client is not aware of the actions and side effects. The reader is advised to consult pharmacological texts for more information on drug action and interaction.

The decreased rate of glomerular filtration common to many older persons, including those in apparently good health, can contribute to drug accumulation in the system. Changes in circulation and liver function also can contribute to the cumulative effects of drugs and the potential of drug toxicity (32). Thus, a dosage which is correct for a 40-year-old person may be too large for an 80-year-old person. Drugs can cause incontinence, urinary retention, gastric bleeding, fluid re- tention, impotency, depression, mental confusion, physical weakness, and many other side effects.

Since older people who see themselves as healthy are often on main- tainence dosages of drugs that control chronic health problems, careful evaluation of all drug intake is important. Moreover, the tendency to believe that there is a drug to cure or to control every ailment can compound the drug interaction possibilities. Consideration of the client's visual acuity and memory is also important in determining if he or she can use medications safely and effectively, whether the drug is prescribed by a physician or is an OTC remedy (33).

Often clients do not think of OTC drugs as medication when they are asked about the medications they take. Recently a client proudly told the author that she only takes one pill a day, her "heart pill." A few visits later, the client casually mentioned that she needs "prune juice in addition to Ex-lax pills" to effect elimination. Careful wording of questions in the client's language is important in complete assessment! Sometimes definitions of terms or examples need to be used to clarify the assessment process for the client.

It is also important for the nurse to work with other health professionals, especially the physician and clinical pharmacist, in assessing the drug status of clients and in providing both individualized and public education on the dangers of drug therapy and the importance of knowledgeable use of required medication.

MODIFYING PHYSICAL ASSESSMENT PARAMETERS TO EVALUATE THE OLDER CLIENT

Introduction

The nurse who examines aging people can expect to find a wide variety of functional and morphological differences that distinguish them from their younger counterparts. It is important that the nurse recognize those differences that represent controllable forces that limit the person's health status. Once these forces are identified, the appropriate teaching and/or referral measures can be taken to modify the effects of age-related changes. In the following section, attempts are made to inform the nurse of both the significance and the range of the various age-related developments so he or she may prioritize the assessment findings.

The Integument

After observation of the general condition of the client's visible skin and hair during initial observation and history taking, a more detailed examination follows in the assessment of each anatomical part or physiological system. Throughout the entire physical assessment it should be remembered that chronological age and the associated morphological and functional changes vary in their correlation from person to person. These age-related alterations follow genetically and environmentally influenced timetables that are unique to each person.

The nurse can expect to see several natural skin changes that accompany the hormonal and physiological changes of aging. One inevitable skin change is wrinkling. The dermis or corium layer gradually thins, and there is a concomitant change in its usual ratio of collagen to elastin protein fibers (34). This alteration is evident in the skin's slowed recoil from stretching, a factor that may invalidate the skin-tenting test for the degree of hydration when applied to the older client. In addition, subcutaneous fat diminishes with age, and the depth of the wrinkles is accentuated. With smaller amounts of subcutaneous fatty tissue, the aged person, especially the fair-skinned one, will appear to have rather transparent skin. This is particularly true for skin on the dorsa of the hands and feet and around the eyes. Unfortunately, with these morphological changes the skin has lost some of its original ability to serve as a protective barrier against external injury, and the elderly client will bruise more easily.

The nurse may also see pigmentary changes. Lentigines, also known as age, or liver spots, are brown macules frequently seen on the faces and dorsal surfaces of the hands of elderly whites. These lesions are nonpathognomonic but may be of moderate cosmetic concern to the aging client. They are believed to be of hormonal origin and are exacerbated by exposure to sunlight. Larger areas of brown pigmentation seen on the lower legs are usually the sequelae of diminished venous return from the lower extremities. The red blood cells, slowed in their return to the heart, leach out of the vascular bed and escape into the surrounding interstitial spaces. In breaking down, their hemoglobin content converts to hemosiderin, a ferric oxide pigment that stains the surrounding tissues. With these findings, efforts should be made to determine the client's awareness of measures to increase venous return. Further inspection of the skin may reveal other age-related lesions known as seborrheic keratoses, or more commonly, keratotic warts (35). These proliferations of the stratum corneum, or outermost layer of the skin, are usually found on the face, neck, or torso of the elderly person. They are raised, and vary in size and degree of pigmentation, but characteristically exhibit a cauliflower-like texture. Like lentigines, they have no clinical significance unless their location causes repeated injury. In such cases they should be surgically removed. Keratotic warts found near the scalp and under binding areas of belts, bras, and girdles are those most likely to be traumatized.

Skin tags are often seen. These are small, stemmed projections of flesh on the softer skin of the eyelids, neck, or around the axillae. They may or may not be pigmented. They, too, are no cause for concern but should be protected from injury.

A clinically important age-related condition is actinic keratosis. The elderly client with a considerable history of outdoor employment or leisure activity merits particular attention given to assessment of sun-exposed areas such as hands, ears, face, and neck. These lesions are plaques of scaly texture that vary widely in their color. Actinic keratoses of the lip usually appear white and opaque, while similar lesions on the backs of hands may be pigmented. The nurse finding what appears to be an actinic keratotic lesion should query the client about its duration and about any noticeable changes. A thickening and inflammation may herald a malignant change, and the client should be referred to a physician for future evaluation through biopsy. Since solar involvement in this type of lesion is likely, the client must be cautioned to wear protective clothing and to use sunscreen preparations prescribed by the physician.

Inspection of the skin of lower extremities may also reveal ecchymoses or bruises, which were not reported during the history. These leg injuries may be the result of impaired motor or sensory neurological function. If a sensory deficit exists, the client is not likely to notice the tenderness normally experienced during healing, and he or she may believe the injury to have healed completely. In addition, the bruised area might not be easily seen by the client in the course of daily bathing and dressing. At any rate, such unreported bruising should mandate later inclusion of the appropriate neurological tests.

Finally, palpation of the skin reveals a reduction in perspired moisture and seborrheic lubrication. The skin feels drier and exhibits a fish-scale, or ichthyotic, appearance. Palpation of these extremely dry areas may elicit mild desquamation, and the nurse may see powdery flakes against dark clothing. The client may complain of chronic itching over these areas, especially during the winter.

The elderly client's nails grow more slowly and display more evident vertical ridges. These alterations are believed to be due to a decrease in the keratin protein needed for strong nail matrix. The toenails of the elderly are particularly prone to onchymycoses, or fungal infection. This is probably due to decreased circulation to the nailbeds of the lower extremities. The involved nails (usually on the great toe) will be noticeably thickened and will appear opaquely yellow. This condition usually responds favorably to antibiotic therapy.

Scalp and body hair also undergo variation with aging. The most striking change is loss of hair pigment, or graying. This is another inevitable age change, although the onset and amount of graying varies tremendously among people. In addition to graying, the hairs of both the scalp and body become fewer in number. This is true for both sexes, and may augment any genetic balding forces already in effect. Postmenopausal women who have inherited traits for the male pattern of baldness from both parents may themselves have noticeable hair loss over frontoparietal areas. The examiner should remember that such hair loss can represent a severe emotional problem for the elderly woman in that the valuation of her "crowning glory" is not relinquished with age.

The Eye and Vision

Normal aging is expected to result in certain structural changes in the eye. Fortunately, not all these changes affect the elderly client's vision adversely. Arcus senilis is one of these harmless changes. This results as certain lipid substances are laid down within the corneal epithelium. A thin, bluish-gray ring appears close to the corneal limbus and is visible against the pigments of the iris. As is the case with other lipid-associated conditions, arcus senilis may have genetic determinents, and many aged persons will never develop it.

The iris may also undergo alterations in its appearance. In some people the usually regular distribution of pigment changes and scattered light brown patches appear. However, this change in no way compromises the iris' ability to regulate pupil size in response to light or in accommodation to distance.

A third innocuous change involves the development of pingueculae, or thickened areas of the bulbar conjunctiva. These yellowish papules initially develop on the nasal side of the eye but may appear later on the temporal aspect. At first sight, these lesions appear to interfere with smooth closure of the eyelid, but actually they present no problems, and the client is usually unaware of them.

Other age-related eye conditions may be of clinical importance. Among these are entropion and ectropion. Entropion, or inward turning of the lower lid, and ectropion, the outward turning of the lower lid, are sequelae of loss of tonicity of the orbicularis oculi muscles. When entropion is present, the cornea is prone to repeated irritation, and it may eventually erode. Close inspection is needed to determine whether the lower lashes have scratched the corneal surface. Ectropion causes irritation of the palpebral and bulbar conjuntivae, which become continually exposed to the drying conditions of the external environment. Both lid changes are surgically correctable.

Age-related changes within the lens of the eye may cause visual problems. One of the constituents of the lens, an insoluble albuminoid protein, increases in quantity along with a yellow pigment. The lens becomes slightly less transparent and considerably less elastic (36).

This loss of lens elasticity is termed presbyopia. The client finds that it becomes increasingly difficult for his eyes to accommodate to an object held close at hand. Actually, the punctum proximium, or closest point to which the eyes can accommodate to produce a clear image, increases in distance, and the person may compensate by holding reading material at an arm's length. Convex lenses are the appropriate corrective measure.

As the soluble proteins of the lens are lost and transparency decreases, the refractive index of the lens increases proportionally, and the person suffers loss of visual acuity. This opacification process is called cataract formation. Certain people will become only mildly myopic or nearsighted, while others will form cataracts to a degree where the transmission of light is so reduced that partial blindness ensues. The myopsis of cataract origin may become evident to the client when he finds his presbyotic reading glasses no longer necessary. At the same time, he finds that distant objects become hazy, and that distance lenses are needed to produce clear images.

Dense cataracts can be seen by the examiner without visual instruments. They appear white against the pupillary opening. Less extreme cataract formation may be visualized using the opthalmoscope. If present, these lesions cast dark brown shadows against the reddish pigments of the retina. The ophthalmoscope beam will also cast the shadow of the ciliary muscles of the iris against the retina, and care must be taken not to confuse this with lens opacification. The ophthalmologist will determine the course of cataract therapy, whether surgical or refractive.

The Ear and Hearing

As certain people age, otosclerosis, or a dystrophy of the bony labyrinth of the middle ear, may affect conduction hearing. When the process continues to the point at which one of the ossicles (usually the stapes) becomes ankylosed or fixed, vibrations to the cochlea are impeded and deafness results. Otosclerotic hearing impairment is most frequently detected during the second and third decades of life, yet many years may pass before complete ankylosis and deafness ensues. A small number of persons having otosclerotic changes within the middle ear may never develop an appreciable hearing loss, yet others may have such extensive dystrophy that the inner ear or cochlea is involved. At such a stage, the person would experience sensorineural hearing loss compounded by conduction difficulties. Otosclerotic hearing loss is more common among women and also has a higher incidence among aging whites than for members of the other races. The nurse will usually find this type of hearing loss to be bilateral and symmetrical.

A sensorineural hearing change linked with the aging process is known as presbycusis. This involves the gradual loss in the client's ability to perceive certain sounds. While the exact mechanism by which presbycusis develops is unknown, two possible etiologies have been proposed. The first suggests a loss in the number of sound-sensing neurons within the spiral ganglion of the cochlear branch of the auditory nerve (37). Another possibility could involve an atrophy of the vascular stria or microcirculation of the organ of Corti in the inner ear (38). The first sounds to become difficult to hear are those in the high-frequency range. These are the consonant sounds in the spoken language.

Since the ear functions both in hearing and in the maintenance of balance, it is not unexpected that age-related change within this structure may contribute to the higher incidence of falling in the elderly. It has been proposed that difficulties in maintaining balance may relate to the loss of microscopic clumps of crystals (otoliths) within the inner ear (39). These structures have been observed to grow in number and size from fetal life to young adulthood. Thereafter, they begin to display signs of dissolution and may disappear altogether by age of 70.

The Nose and Oral Cavity

Regarding age-related changes of the oral tissues, it is particularly important to remember the strong influence that environmental factors play in their development. In many cases, environmental elements such as foods, mineral deposits in drinking water, tobacco and alcohol use, extended drug therapies, and ultraviolet radiation may be more closely linked to oral disease than is aging per se or any genetic predisposition. Often, the dose-response ratio of these environmental elements becomes significant only after the sixth or seventh decade of life and is mistakenly viewed as idiopathic degeneration due to aging.

A particular example is evident in the occurrence of dental caries among Americans of all ages and in the frequent edentulousness of Americans over 65 years of age. Many people believe that teeth are simply temporary anatomical blocks of enamel that are meant to decay and then to be removed (40). Little speculation is given, among the general population, as to whether any intervening factors exist such as diet, oral hygiene, and heredity. Unfortunately, the myth is perpetuated that tooth decay, loss of teeth, and aging go hand in hand.

The extant teeth of the aged person will show signs of wear. Even in cases of good occlusion, or alignment of the chewing surfaces, the enamel will have worn away, leaving the yellowish-colored dentin visible. This is especially evident in the lower incisors. Vertical cracks in the enamel of the incisors are due to the individual's exposure to extremes of temperature encountered in hot and cold beverages and subfreezing weather. These fissures extend no deeper than the enamel layer and present no added access for cariogenic bacteria.

The remaining teeth of the elderly person may exhibit more of the neck portion because of the loss of the supporting bone structure. This appearance is indicative of periodontal disease and gives rise to the pejorative description of aging, that is, appearing "a little long in the tooth." Like tooth decay, periodontal disease (i.e., disease involving gingivae and supporting bone) is strongly associated with poor oral hygiene (41) and should not be viewed merely as a consequence of growing older. In such cases, teeth usually reveal deposits of tartar over the neck portions where they present a chronic source of irritation to the gums. The inflammatory response of the gingivae is followed by a resorption of the teeth-supporting alveolar ridges. Gradually, the teeth loosen and fall out. In conjunction with examination of the teeth the nurse can provide health teaching to motivate the client to practice effective hygienic measures since these will prevent or control the process in the majority of cases.

Bone loss in certain people continues after the loss of all the teeth necessitating repeated refitting of dentures. Ill-fitting plates are another source of gingival irritation. The nurse should inspect the alveolar ridges under the dentures for friction lesions and attempt to locate the causative area on the prosthesis. The client should be advised of the need for refitting by the dentist.

Occasionally, the older client will complain of lessened ability to taste certain substances. The smaller papillae, or taste buds, on the anterior portion of the tongue are known to atrophy with aging, but this loss of taste may actually be due to changes in the ability to perceive smells. Since the nose plays a large part in the interpretation of the more complex tastes, that is, those beyond the basic sensations of sweet, sour, salty, and bitter, the client may be experiencing hyposmia or a desensitization to certain odors. Because the actual mechanism of scent receptor function is not fully understood, the fact that the elderly experience some degree of hyposmia has been observed but not explained. Theories have been postulated that there may be changes in specific molecular receptor sites that would perhaps influence selective absorption of various molecular (scent) stimuli (42).

The Respiratory System

The aging process has been linked to various alterations in respiratory function. These appear to be due to a loss of elasticity of the tissues immediately surrounding the alveolar sacs (42). This loss of elasticity affects the older client's pulmonary compliance, or the ratio of the lung volume increase to the unit increase in intra-alveolar pressure. This means that as the pressure builds within the alveolar sacs during inspiration, the lung as a whole is slower and less able to respond by fully collapsing during expiration. Age-related skeletal deformities of the thorax may compound disturbances of pulmonary compliance (44). Such losses of tissue elasticity also result in an increase in the client's residual air volume, or the quantity of air left in the lungs after the most forceful exhalation. In addition, there is a decrease in the inspiratory reserve volume, that is, the quantity of air that can be taken in over and beyond the tidal flow exchanged during normal breathing. This, in turn, reduces the elderly person's total lung capacity, or the maximum volume to which his lungs will expand with the greatest possible inspiratory effort (45). The older client takes shallower, more frequent breaths than his younger counterpart.

Unfortunately, this loss of parenchymal elasticity alters the gas diffusing mechanism of the respiratory membrane. The slackened alveolar walls effect a sac volume increase, which, in turn, causes a drop in intra-alveolar pressure (46). As the intra-alveolar pressure falls below a certain point, the sacs in the lower lung fields close out of synchrony with those in the apices. In a well, younger person, the alveoli of the lung bases are small, and those in the apices have greater diameter (47). This size relationship in the older client is reversed, causing his lungs to have their greatest air volumes at the bases. However, the greatest quantity of diffused, exchanged air will be found in the older client's upper lung fields since these alveoli are smaller and faster closing than those in the slackened lower sacs. Consequently, most of the elderly person's ventilation occurs in the apices despite the fact that his lungs have the highest degree of blood flow in the gravity-dependent bases. The result is an uneven distribution of ventilation evidenced by decreased levels of arterial P_aO_2. (48).

All these changes progressively lower total pulmonary function, and the older person often becomes more likely to develop non-age-related lung conditions. He or she becomes increasingly more vulnerable to the hazards posed by smoking and by breathing polluted air. Weather or climatic conditions resulting in high air concentrations of sulfur and nitrogen oxide, carbon monoxide, hydrocarbon, and particulate emissions are especially dangerous to the aging person. In addition, increased pulmonary function causes the elderly person who is "easily winded" to be less likely to engage in needed physical activity.

Cardiovascular System

Reduced cardiac efficiency among older persons with no previous history of heart dysfunction seems to stem from certain mechanical disturbances of the myocardial tissue. These changes have been postulated to result from a decrease in the swelling property of myocardial proteins and have been linked to a loss of heart muscle elasticity (49). A decrease in elasticity reduces ventricular compliance, and more time is needed for the right ventricle to fill with blood during diastole (50). This, through homeostatic mechanisms, reduces the older person's cardiac output, or the amount of blood pumped by the left ventricle each minute. This reduction occurs in order to reestablish the balance between the blood volumes of venous return and cardiac output. Gradually, over long periods of time, the amount of blood pumped by the left ventricle may become sufficiently reduced to cause the heart's autoregulator to prolong contraction time, or systole. At rest, the older client's heart rate is usually slower than that of a younger adult. A lowered cardiac output also indicates that less oxygen will be available for the increased tissue requirements caused by prolonged strenuous exercise. The older client should be advised to recognize his fatigue-response as an indicator of overtaxing physical activity. Extended exercise at straining levels, such as shoveling snow or lifting heavy objects, is likely to result in temporary or prolonged ischemia of skeletal or cardiac muscle.

Age-related changes in the nature of heart sounds are often noticed on auscultation. The older person's heart valves may develop fibrotic or nodular areas (51). When the aortic and pulmonic valves develop fibrotic changes to the point of effecting incomplete closure, murmurs may be heard on auscultation.

Blood pressure norms for the aging population have been an area of some uncertainty. Previously it was believed that pressure norms for well elderly preople could be expected to be somewhat higher than those for younger people. This was thought to result from decreased effectiveness of pressure-sensitive receptor cells, situated in the carotid sinus (52). Elderly men with blood pressures below 160/100 mmHg and women with pressures below 170/90 mmHg were considered normotensive for their age (53). More recent evidence shows that one can expect only a slight elevation in systolic pressure and little or no rise in diastolic figures with advancing age (54). This suggests that the norms established for younger adults may also apply to the healthy aged population. In agreement were the blood pressure means published by the United States Department of Health, Education and Welfare for a survey population of 6,000 persons aged 18 to 74 years. Blood pressure norms for men 60 to 74 years of age ranged from 110/70 mmHg to 148.4/85.6 mmHg; norms for women of the same age category ranged from 105/65 mmHg to 148.4/85.6 mmHg (55).

The Musculoskeletal System

The older client is likely to experience a reduction in the size of skeletal muscles despite the fact that some physical exercise is part of his or her daily regime. The diameters of the individual muscle fibers decrease as they gradually lose the constituent myofibrils. This is an expected development since older clients rightly avoid engaging in the forceful, resistive, or isometric exercise necessary for muscular hypertrophy, or new myofibril formation. It has been estimated that muscle building (myofibril formation) is unlikely to occur unless the muscle contracts to at least 75% of its maximum tension. Weaker activity, that is, exercise appropriate for aged persons, even for prolonged periods, will probably not result in muscle hypertrophy or in a perpetuation of earlier levels of muscle mass. Recognizing that muscle size is apt to decrease with age, the nurse should ascertain that the decrease results in a gradual, symmetric and essentially nonlimiting loss of motive power for the client.

A loss of bone tissue density without a disruption of the usual calcium salt-to-collagen-fiber ratio appears to be an age-related phenomenon (56). The collagen component of bone gives the skeletal parts tensile strength, while the calcium compounds allow for compressional stress. When both components gradually diminish proportionally, the bones become more vulnerable to bending as well as to impact stresses. Fractures can result from performing previously innocuous activities. To some degree this loss of bone tissue is probably related to the rather sedentary activity levels of certain older persons of both sexes, since osteoblastic activity responds proportionally to the compressional burden of the skeleton during exercise. In addition, bone tissue density changes appear to be aggravated by estrogen diminutions in postmenopausal women since this hormone is known to stimulate osteoblastic activity (57). Moreover, chronically low dietary intake of calcium among elderly women has been shown to compound age-related hormonal effects to produce moderate to severe bone loss. Fortunately, some studies reveal that this loss of bone structure and its associated risk of fracture can be slowed or reversed. A daily calcium intake of 800 to 1,000 mg of calcium appears to be necessary to maintain optimal bone health in postmenopausal women (56, 58). Since this amount represents the calcium in a quart of whole or skim milk, it is unlikely that this requirement will be met without tablet supplements prescribed by a physician. This is also true for the older client who must restrict fluids and/or animal fats in the diet for therapeutic reasons.

Loss of bone density eventually causes skeletal alterations. Among the more obvious is a loss of height, which occurs predominately within the cervical to sacral spinal area. The anterior to posterior curvature of this section of the spinal column becomes more flexed and the older client develops a kyphotic or round shouldered appearance. When this anterior to posterior spinal deformity also has lateral components, that is, kyphoscoliosis, a shifting of the apex of the heart may disassociate the apical impulse from its usual thoracic landmarks. Similarly, the trachea may also be deviated by skeletal changes from midline.

Most elderly people develop some degree of osteoarthritis (59). This is characterized by a gradual breakdown of joint cartilage and by a hypertrophy of bone tissue at the osteochondral margins. The resulting stiffness and mild pain on motion is almost always relieved by resting the affected joint. However, the avoidance of certain recreational activities may be particularly frustrating to the aging client who has recently adopted them to replace others currently proscribed. Yet, continued overuse of affected joints is likely to exacerbate mobility problems. This age-related type of arthritis produces only a minor amount of joint swelling, but when the digits are involved, the client may have difficulty in performing fine motor movements. Rings worn below swollen joints may be impossible to slide off.

The Neurological System

As a person reaches middle age, he or she begins to lose a small percentage of brain cells. It might be assumed, therefore, that eventually, in old age, various cerebral functions would become noticeably impaired. This does not appear to be the case, however, perhaps because neurons within certain brain centers have functional overlap or duplication with those in other brain areas. This could allow for some degree of compensation for functional losses.

Functional changes are known to result, however, when enzymatic activity at neuromuscular junctions decreases. Actually, aging of the neuromuscular apparatus results in various interrelated physiological changes, each of which lessens the older person's reaction time. When a nerve impulse is transmitted to the neuromuscular junction, acetylcholine is released by the end plate of the nerve fiber into the synapse or space between it and the skeletal muscle fiber. The enzyme remains active there for approximately two milliseconds until aggregates of cholinesterase from the muscle fiber render it inactive. During that short period, acetylcholine excites the muscle fiber by effecting a rapid increase in the permeability of the muscle fiber membrane to sodium ions. As acetylcholine is hydrolyzed by cholinesterase, this permeability to sodium returns to the resting level. In this creation of a reversible sodium conductivity, acetylcholine is said to cause an action potential. The period of time associated with establishment of the action potential is longer in older persons (60) and suggests a delayed return of sodium permeability to resting stages and additional time requirements for re-excitation of the motoneuron. This, in turn, affects the speed at which nerve impulses are conducted along nerve fibers, gradually causing the older person to experience slowed reaction times, which may interfere with his or her ability to perform certain tasks smoothly or safely. For example, for some older people, driving may become an inordinately challenging situation in which slowed response can clearly be a liability.

The elderly person's ability to recall recently learned information may also lessen in the process of aging. The fact that long-range memory in the aged often remains unaffected in the presence of short-term memory deficits may be explained by physiological and site differences between the two thought processes. Recent memory is believed to involve an electrochemical perpetuation of the original stimulus within the neurons of the cortex. The particular brain area excited by the stimulus continues to emit rhythmic action potentials. While these electrical impulses continue, they provide instant recall of the initial sensation or thought. If the impulses are perpetuated beyond a critical period, their pattern becomes fixed, and the originating stimulus may be remembered days or years later. In support of this theory of memory, it is known that any factor causing a disruption of brain function, such as seizure or trauma, prevents fixation of recent memory. Elimination of the disturbance does not result in memory of events immediately precedent to it. In the elderly the "disturbance" is believed to be a chronically diminished oxygen supply, which may continually interfere with memory fixation. It is also believed that certain areas of the brain that serve as long-range memory depots are not as sensitive to hypoxic states as are recent memory sites. For this reason, it has been postulated that memory transference from one site to another may occur as part of the fixation process. Therefore, while recent memory lapses are not uncommon among the well elderly population, long-term recall, by contrast, remains quite adequate unless affected by an underlying pathologic condition.

Mild memory and intellectual dysfunction may be evident in the older person's inability to recall breakfast items and/or to carry out calculations such as determining the number of quarters in $5.50. Severe impairment may cause an inability to recall one's age or date of birth. The nurse should remember that a client's inability to supply age or birthday may not be significant if evidence of higher functioning is given, such as correctly adding or subtracting serial sevens or solving difficult money problems. In such cases, these inabilities may be due to inattention or hearing impairment (61).

Mood assessment in the elderly is often difficult because of the similarity between the degree and symptoms associated with depression and those related to healthful aging. Loss of energy, decline of appetite, and a variety of sleep disturbances may all be consequences of the aging process without heralding either physical or psychological disease. At the same time, these symptoms may be suggestive of depressive states requiring therapy. Establishing the recent onset of such developments will cue the nurse to include additional questions more diagnostic of depression in the interview. Client responses to such questions as "Are you no longer interested in doing things you once enjoyed?" or "Do you find yourself sitting for hours really feeling down?" should be evaluated along with nonverbal indicators such as posture, gesticulation, attentiveness, and hygiene. While suicide may be proportionally more frequent among teens and young adults, the older client may also be considered less able to adapt to developmental stresses such as loss of spouse, chronic illness, or forced dependency. Once evidence of suicidal intent is elicited, the nurse should make the appropriate referrals.

There are also peripheral neurological changes among elderly people. Deep tendon reflexes, with the possible exception of the Achilles tendon reflex, should be present as in younger clients. Often, eliciting the ankle jerk response can be done only through the examiner's use of reinforcement techniques that may cause the older client to lose his balance and fall. Consequently, failure to elicit the ankle jerk bilaterally when the client is sitting or reclining should not be taken as evidence of its total absence.

Examination of the sensory component of the neurological system of a well older person should evaluate sensations of light touch, pain, vibration, and muscle-joint position. Once light touch sensation is established, testing for simultaneous sensation extinction can be done to reveal temporal lobe lesions. The results of these sensory evaluations should not differ greatly from those conducted with well younger clients. The nurse can expect the vibration sense to be absent or diminished bilaterally on the ankle and/or toe joints of older people because of degenerative changes in peripheral nerves. A more significant finding would be the absence of vibratory sense at midshin level since this would suggest peripheral neuropathies not solely attributable to the aging process. Pain sense tested through pin pricking may be obscured by callous formation on the toes or finger pads, therefore, it may be necessary to apply slightly more pressure to elicit the pain response in the older client.

Genitourinary System

The aging process may be linked with functional and morphological changes in the kidneys. The kidneys are known to decrease in size as the person ages. This loss of tissue appears to be confined more to cortical than to medullary areas, and it is thought that this size reduction is a consequence of diffuse vascular changes (ischemic scarring) rather than to localized areas of pyelonephritic scar formation (62). This gradual loss of renal tissue does not appear to result in functional impairment since the kidneys appear to have a large functional reserve. Less than half the usual number of nephrons can eliminate waste products from the body if average amounts of protein and electrolytes are ingested.

Functional changes do occur when an older client's cardiac output is reduced because of myocardial alterations. The renal fraction, which amounts to approximately 21% of the cardiac output, is reduced proportionally, resulting in decreased blood flow through renal arterioles.

Loss of muscle tone in the perineal floor is an age-related cause of stress incontinence in women. In men, urinary problems such as increased frequency and difficulty in starting and stopping the flow of urine may result from prostatic gland hypertrophy.

Pelvic examination of the postmenopausal woman reveals reductions in uterine and cervical size. The vaginal walls become thinner, and quantitative and qualitative changes take place in mucous secretion. Usually no problems result unless the adrenals are unable to supply sufficient estrogen to maintain these tissues after menopause.

In such cases the physician may prescribe estrogen replacements to treat vaginal lesions and/or infections that develop due to tissue friability and alterations in the pH of secretions.

Among the secondary sexual characteristics that also respond to changing hormonal levels postmenopausally are the breasts. Gradually, fat replaces the atrophying glandular tissue and results in a change more related to consistency than to size.

The reproductive tissues of elderly men also respond to lowered levels of hormone production. There is a reduction in testicular size and a concommitant reduction in gametogenesis in the seminiferous tubules. The amount and composition of seminal fluid is altered, due, in part, to changes within the prostate gland. None of these changes should greatly affect potency or fertility.

SUMMARY

Changes in a person's physical status are often more immediately evident than psychosocial changes. Moreover, according to Maslow's hierarchy of needs, physical needs must be satisfied at least minimally before other needs can become preeminent.

Biological theories of aging provide a scientific framework for a realistic view of the physical changes of aging. Considered alone, the physical changes of aging can present a negative outlook. However, certain health practices promote the maintainence of optimum health. These include adequate rest, regular physical activity, and proper nutrition.

Nevertheless, physical changes do occur with aging. Some changes are simply due to the aging process with no pathological ramifications. In assessing the healthy elderly client, the nurse should know which changes are harmless and which may be indicative of disease processes.

A holistic view of a client considers his or her physical status in concert with the psychological, sociological, and cultural components of life.

REFERENCES

1. Hayflick L: Current theories of biological aging. *Federation Proceedings, Federation of American Societies for Experimental Biology* 34: 9–13, 1975.

2. Martin GE, Sprague CA, Epstein CJ: Replicative life-span of cultivated human cells. *Laboratory Investigation* 23:86–92, 1970.
3. Cristofalo VJ: Animal cell cultures as a model system for the study of aging, in Strehler BL (ed): *Advances in Gerontological Research*, vol. 4. New York: Academic Press, 1972.
4. Kohn R: *Principles of Mammalian Aging,* ed 2. Englewood Cliffs, N.J., Prentice-Hall, 1978.
5. Kuhn W: Possible relation between optical activity and aging. *Adv Enzymol* 20:1–30, 1958.
6. Harman D, Heidrick ML, Eddy DE: Free Radical Theory of Aging. *J Am Geriatr Soc* 25:400, 1977.
7. Teller MN: Age changes and immune resistance to cancer, in Strehler BL (ed): *Advances in Gerontological Research*, vol 4. New York, Academic Press, 1972, p 39.
8. Dunn HL: What high level wellness means. *Canadian J Pub Health* 50:447–457, 1959.
9. Stenbeck A, Kumpulamen M, Vauhkonon ML: Illness and health in septuagenarians. *J Gerontol* 33:57–61, 1978.
10. Belloc NB, Breslow L: Relationship of physical health status and health practices. *Prevent Med* 1:409–421, 1972.
11. Sherman ED: Geriatric profile of Thomas Jefferson. *J Amer Geriatr Soc* 25:113, 1977.
12. Goldman R: Rest: its use and abuse in the aged. *J Amer Geriatr Soc* 25:433, 1977.
13. Luce GG: *Current Research on Sleep and Dreams*. Washington DC, US Government Printing Office, 1975.
14. Kales A: Sleep and dreams—recent research on clinical aspects. *Ann Intern Med* 68:1081, 1968.
15. Dement WC: *Some Must Watch While Some Must Sleep*. San Francisco, WH Freeman and Co, 1974.
16. Feinberg I: Changes in sleep cycle patterns with age. *J Psychiatr Res* 10:283–306, 1974.
17. Kraus H: Preservation of physical fitness, in Harris R, Frankel LJ: *Guide to Fitness After Fifty*. New York, Plenum Press, 1977, p 35.
18. Bottiger LE: Regular decline in physical working capacity with age. *Brit Med J* 3:270–271, 1973.
19. Hennekens CH, Rosner B, Jesse MJ, et al: A retrospective study of physical activity and coronary deaths. *Int J Epidemiol* 6:243–246, 1977.
20. Simonson E: Effect of age on work and fatigue—cardiovascular aspects, in Harris R, Frankel LJ: *Guide to Fitness After Fifty*. New York, Plenum Press, 1977, p 55.
21. Devries HA: Physiology of physical conditioning for the elderly, in Harris R and Frankel LJ: *Guide to Fitness After Fifty*. New York, Plenum Press, 1977, p 51.
22. Winick M (ed): *Nutrition and Aging*. New York, John Wiley, 1976.
23. Christakis G (ed): Nutritional assessment in health programs. *Amer J Pub Health* 63: Supplement, 1973.

24. Weg RB: *Nutrition and the Later Years.* Los Angeles, University of Southern California Press, 1978, p 202.
25. Grotkowski ML, Sims LS: Nutritional knowledge, attitudes, and dietary practices of the elderly. *J Am Diet Assoc* 72:499–505, 1978.
26. O'Hanlon P, Kohrs MB: Dietary studies of older Americans. *Am J Clin Nutr,* July 1978, pp 1257–1269.
27. Fisher S, Hendricks DG, Mahoney AW: Nutritional assessment of senior rural Utahns by biochemical and physical measurements. *Am J Clin Nutrea,* April 1978, pp 667–672.
28. Dickerson JWT: Nutrition, aging and the elderly. *Roy Soc Hlth* 98:81–83, 95, April 1978.
29. Templeton CL: Nutrition counseling needs in a geriatric population. *Geriatrics,* April 1978, pp 59–66.
30. Rao DB: Problems of nutrition in the aged. *J Amer Geriatr Soc* 21:362–367, 1973.
31. Lamy PP: The food/drug connection in elderly patients. *Am Pharmacy.* NS18:30–31, 1978.
32. Richey DP: Effects of human aging on drug absorption and metabolism, in Goldman R, Rockstein M (eds): *The Physiology and Pathology of Human Aging.* New York, Academic Press, 1975, pp 59–93.
33. Olson J, Johnson J: Drug misuse among the elderly. *J Gerontol Nurs* 4:11–14, 1978.
34. Demis D, Crounse R, McGuire J, et al: *Clinical Dermatology,* vol 1, sec 1–5. Hagerstown, Md, Harper & Row Publishers, 1979.
35. Selmanowitz V: Cutaneous changes associated with aging. *J Dermatol Surg* 3:628–634, 1977.
36. Klintworth G, Landers M: *The Eye–Structure and Function in Disease.* Baltimore, Md, William & Wilkins Company, 1976.
37. Saxen A, von Fieandt H: Pathologic und Klinik der Altersschwerhorigkeit. *Acta Otolaryngol* suppl 23, 1937, p 1.
38. Johnsson L, Hawkins J: A direct approach to cochlear anatomy and pathology in man. *Arch Otolaryngol* 85:599–613, 1972.
39. Ross MD, et al: Observations on normal and degenerating human otoconia. *Ann Otol, Rhinol Laryngol* 85:310, 1976.
40. Mitchell D, Standish M, Fast T: *Oral Diagnosis and Oral Medicine.* Philadelphia, Lea and Febiger, 1971, p 59.
41. *Selected Dental Findings in Adults by Age, Race and Sex: United States.* Public Health Service Pub, No. 1000, Series II, No. 7, 1960–1962.
42. Barnhardt R: Medical treatment of nasal and sinus diseases, in *Otolaryngology Vol II.* Hagerstown, Md, Harper & Row Publishers. 1977.
43. Dhar S, Shastri SR, Lenora RAK: Aging and the respiratory system. *Med Clin North Am* 60:1121–1139, 1976.
44. Guyton AC: *Basic Human Physiology Normal Function and Mechanisms of Disease.* Philadelphia: WB Saunders Company, 1971, chaps 27, 28.
45. Gelb AE, Zamel N: The effect of aging on lung mechanisms in healthy non-smokers. *Chest* 68:538–541, 1975.

46. Anthonisen NR, et al: Airway closure as a function of age. *Respiratory Physiology* 8:58–65, 1969.
47. Shapiro B: *Clinical Applications of Blood Gases.* Chicago, Year Book Medical Publishers, 1973, chap 7.
48. Sorbini CA, Grassi V, Solinas E, et al: Arterial oxygen tension in relation to age in healthy subjects. *Respirations* 25:3–13, 1968.
49. Kohn RR, Rollerson E: Studies on the mechanism of the age related changes in the swelling ability of human myocardium. *Circ Res* 7:740, 1959.
50. Sebbon C, et al: Ventricular compliance and aging. *Biomedicine* 22:56–61, 1975.
51. Pomerance A: Pathogenesis of senile nodular sclerosis of atrioventricular valves. *Brit Heart J* 28:815, 1966.
52. Frolkis VV, Bezrukov VV, Shevchuk VG: Hemodynamics and its regulation in old age. *Exp Gerontol* 10:251–271, 1975.
53. Masters AM, Lasser RP: Blood pressure elevation in the elderly patient. in Brest AN, Myoer JH (eds): *Hypertension.* Second Hahnemann Symposium on Hypertensive Disease. Lea and Febiger, 1964.
54. Babu TN, et al: What is normal blood pressure in the aged? *Geriatrics* 32:73–76, 1977.
55. *National Health Survey: Blood Pressure of Persons 18–74 Years in the U.S. 1971–1972.* Rockville, Md, National Center for Health Statistics, US Department of Health Education and Welfare, 1975.
56. Alabanese A: Calcium nutrition in the elderly: maintaining bone health to minimize fracture risk. *Postgrad Med.* 73:167–172, 1978.
57. Urist MR: Osteoporosis in post menopausal women. *Medical Folio* 3:1, 1971.
58. US Department of Agricultural Research Services: *Dietary Levels of Household.* Washington DC, US Government Printing Office, 1968.
59. Krupp M and Chatton M: *Current Medical Diagnosis and Treatment.* Los Altos, Calif, Lange Medical Publications, 1975, chap 13.
60. Frolkis VV, Martynenko OA, Zamostyan VP: Aging of the neuromuscular apparatus. *Gerontology* 22:244–279, 1976.
61. Caird FI, Judge TG: *Assessment of the Elderly Patient.* Kent, England, Pitman Medical Publishing Company, 1974.
62. Griffiths GJ, Robinson KB, et al: Loss of renal tissue in the elderly. *Brit J Radiol* 49:111–117, 1976.

ANNOTATED BIBLIOGRAPHY

Goldman R, Rockstein, M (eds): *The Physiology and Pathology of Human Aging.* New York, Academic Press, 1975.
  A symposium publication by various contributors covering a broad range

of topics including some specific disease processes in the elderly, drug metabolism in the elderly, sleep and aging, and sexuality in the elderly.

Harris R, Frankel LJ: *Guide to Fitness After Fifty*. New York, Plenum Press, 1977.

A collection of papers by various contributors that gives research data, an historical background, and some practical guides to physical exercise programs for older persons. Particular emphasis is on the importance of the role of the health professional in the education and motivation of persons to increase their physical activity so their physical health can be maintained and/or improved.

Kohn, RR: *Principles of Mammalian Aging,* ed 2. Englewood Cliffs, NJ, Prentice-Hall, 1978.

A well-written review of research on the biology of aging that focuses primarily on the collagen cross-linkage theory of biological aging.

Winick, M (ed): *Nutrition and Aging*. New York, John Wiley and Sons, 1976.

Fourth in a series of volumes on nutrition and persons of different ages. Reports on research about nutrition and the biology of aging, physiological aspects of nutrition, and nutrition-related diseases that older persons sometimes experience.

chapter four
psychological health
in the second half of life

I relive so many poignant experiences, brief and fleeting, the imprints of which lie deep and clear in my heart. I have outgrown my morbid sensitiveness and have broken away from the bondage of my vanities. . . .

Pain and struggle have not been lacking, but on the whole, my life has been a rich experience. As I travel on toward the unknown, the winds of change sweep through vast areas, and I am aware of the death agonies of an obsolete civilization. While my confidence in many of my old beliefs is crumbling, I cling to the belief that the destiny of man points upward.

When the bell tolls for me, I shall go willingly, with no bitterness, but with tenderness toward my fellow travelers on my long journey.

Polly Francis, age 91
The Washington Post, March 16, 1975

OUTLINE

DEFINING PSYCHOLOGICAL HEALTH

The psychology of each person is an important component of the whole being. Human psychology is complex and multidimensional; it can be viewed from behavioral perspectives or from a person's internal frame of reference. To most completely account for the multidimensionality of psychological health, a combination assessment of overt behavioral characteristics and a person's own description of his internal frame of reference is most helpful. Observation for congruity between these two components provides information about the client's psychological health, but the observer needs to be careful that she or he does not project personal standards of psychological health on to the client.

Use of both objective and subjective data about psychological health is especially important when the client is an older person, since aging is a changing process and the methods used to assess the psychological health of a child or a young adult might give a limited perspective of an older person. The nurse's beliefs and values about aging can easily influence interpretation of objective observations, therefore, the subjective perceptions of the client about his health status are essential. In addition, the client who is older usually has a larger experience repertoire than does the nurse and may, therefore, have a broader conceptual base for defining "health." The use of the phrases "perception of his own health status" and "beliefs about whether he is healthy" are consistent with this idea. Usually the client who believes he or she is healthy will also have overt behaviors that an observer would describe as characteristic of a healthy status.

Many studies have been done to identify what successful or healthy aging is from a psychological perspective. Studies that take into account both the behavioral and self-report components of psychological health assessment are those done by Neugarten and her associates. They have identified five components of life satisfaction: 1) zest versus apathy, 2) resolution and fortitude, 3) congruence between desired and achieved goals, 4) positive self concept, and 5) mood tone (see Fig. 6) (1).

Zest can be described as enthusiasm and personal involvement in activities that provide meaning to life. *Apathy*, on the other end of the continuum, means listlessness, lack of energy, and boredom in relation to any activities, either alone or with others.

Resolution and fortitude are described as personal assumption of responsibility for life and actions as opposed to passively allowing things to happen to self. Resolution and fortitude are consistent with Erikson's idea of ego integrity and Maslow's description of a person who is self-actualized.

Goal congruence is a category used to evaluate whether a person's goals have been achieved as planned and desired. A low score (see Fig. 6) in this category involves a person feeling that he or she has not used available opportunities in a satisfactory manner. Expressions of regret would signify goal incongruence.

Self-concept includes physical, psychological, and social expressions of self. People who care about how they appear to others, who are

Apathy	(1)	Zest
Passivity	(2)	Resolution/fortitude
Unfulfilled goals	(3)	Goals achieved
Negative self-concept	(4)	Positive self-concept
Bitter	(5)	Happy
Low	Score	High

Figure 6. Life satisfaction components (1 to 5) on a continuum correlated with life satisfaction score.

comfortable with who they are, and who enjoy their relationship with others would score high on self-concept. Someone who cares little about personal grooming, feels incompetent in his or her actions, and perceives self as a burden on others would be described as having a low self-concept.

The *mood tone* component has a high rating for the person who is optimistic and generally happy, who can see the good in self and others, and who finds pleasure in life. Conversely, the person who is bitter, pessimistic, and frequently irritable would be described as rating low on the mood tone component.

More than a decade ago, Havighurst (2) pointed out that there are two prevailing theories of successful aging; activity theory and disengagement theory. Those who support the activity theory see older persons as essentially the same in relation to psychological and social needs as when they were younger. For instance, a person who is aging successfully remains active and involved in life.

The disengagement theory supports the idea that there comes a time in the older person's life when he or she and society initiate a decrease in social interaction and activity. This theory states that this disengagement process is accepted, and sometimes desired, by the older person.

Research has revealed that both types of aging occur, and a more effective approach to the question would be to see it as a continuum (see Fig. 7). Studies show that life satisfaction correlates highly with active persons whose personalities are integrated or armoured as compared with less active, passive, and unintegrated personality types (3). Although there are some exceptions, research of primarily healthy older populations supports the activity theory of successful aging.

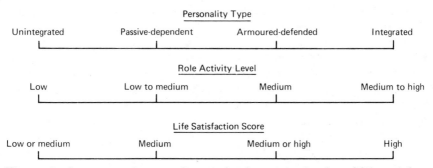

Figure 7. Continuua of personality type, role activity level, and life satisfaction score. (Figure is based on data from the Kansas City Study of Adult Life.)

Since aging is a process of change, a developmental approach is helpful in establishing assessment guidelines for psychological health in the older person. This is not to say that behaviorists, cognitivists, and others have not contributed to the current body of psychological knowledge. Rather, developmental psychology provides a systematic structure for unifying the body of knowledge as it applies to the mental health of older persons.

Furthermore, a philosophical orientation that considers the whole person to be a unique and important entity provides a meaningful base on which to build a unifying frame of reference in psychological assessment.

PSYCHOLOGICAL DEVELOPMENT IN AGING

Erikson's theory of development is based on his observations of clients in his basically psychoanalytic view of psychology. However, Maslow, who comes from the humanistic school of psychology, and is seen as a founder of the humanistic school of psychology in America, lists a hierarchy of needs. Although these needs are seen as basic to a human being at any stage of development, a certain amount of synthesis can occur when Maslow and Erikson's theories are used together to assess the older adult. Furthermore, a blending of a developmental and a humanistic view contributes to a holistic approach.

Much of early psychological study, both developmental and analytic, dealt more with child development than with adult development. Examples are the work of Freud, Piaget, and others.

Looking at Maslow's hierarchy of needs (see Table 6), it is easy to see that people in any developmental stage must have their basic needs met. Basic needs are physiological, security, and belonging needs, and the need for self-esteem. Physiological, safety and belonging needs are important to a newborn infant, a school-aged child, and an adult. As the child grows, his self-esteem needs surface when physiological, safety, and belonging needs are met. Metaneeds (self-actualization) in Maslow's hierarchy, are more likely present, at least in a conscious way, for persons who are approaching or have achieved adulthood or maturity. In the category of self-actualization, a certain amount of similarity exists between Erikson's and Peck's outline of the development of middle age and older adults.

If it is true that Americans often lack purpose in old age (4), then ambivalence and negative attitudes about aging can be readily un-

Table 6. Maslow's Motivation (Need) Hierarchy

I. Deficiency needs (basic needs)
  A. Fundamental needs
    1. Physiological
      a. Oxygen
      b. Circulation
      c. Water
      d. Rest
      e. Nutrition
      f. Elimination
      g. Mobility
      h. Sex
  B. Intermediate needs
    1. Security
      a. Physical
      b. Psychological
      c. Financial
    2. Belonging
      a. Love
      b. Acceptance
      c. Understanding
    3. Self-esteem
      a. Self-respect (privacy)
      b. Self-esteem (personal hygiene)
      c. Self-worth
      d. Recognition
II. Growth needs (metaneeds)
  A. Self-actualization
    1. Justice
    2. Goodness
    3. Beauty
    4. Order
    5. Unity

derstood. In spite of much coverage of aging in the media, in various professional endeavors, and in government-sponsored programs, ambivalence and reticence about aging pervades American society. Because of this, an examination of the psychological aspects of aging from a theoretical model, which is developmental in design, provides a meaningful approach and increased optimism about the aging process. Peck's expansion of Erikson's eight stages of man provides such a theoretical model.

DEVELOPMENTAL STAGES OF ADULTHOOD

Peck divides middle age into four stages and old age into three stages, which "may occur in different time sequence, for different individuals" (5). These stages are pictured in Figure 8.

It is important to note at this point that in none of these dichotomies is the best on one side and the worst on the other side. Instead, a balance of the two dichotomous components portrays a more holistic perspective of human adult development. Here the use of a continuum construct would show that most people fall somewhere along the line between the two dichotomies rather than at either extreme.

Middle Age

Valuing Wisdom Versus Valuing Physical Power

The importance of maintaining physical health and stamina should not be disregarded, as was pointed out in Chapter 3. However, as a person ages, the developmental tasks that are faced in the middle years involve prioritizing of value systems. From a holistic standpoint, therefore, a person's life experiences, his decision-making abilities, and the insights that he has gained from living a certain number of years can decrease the importance of prowess, strength, attractiveness, and beauty. This is not to say that an awareness of how one looks is not still important, but it is not the all consuming force that it was during adolescence.

Wisdom is not simply intellectual ability. Rather, it is a more holistic concept that includes experiential and intuitional knowledge and conceptual skills and their application. Some of the writings about "middle-age crises" relate very closely to the struggle to achieve a meaningful and liberating balance between the values of wisdom and physical power.

People who are cognizant of who they are as whole persons rather than who they are as physical persons can be said to have achieved this balance. This can happen more readily when, in Maslow's terms, people's basic needs have been and are being met, and they have achieved a certain amount of self-actualization through their own creative efforts.

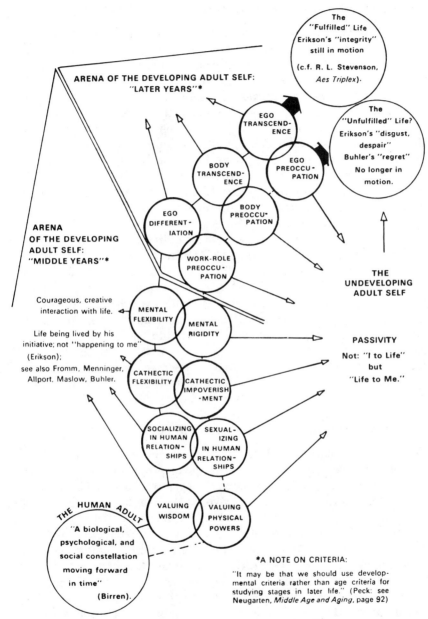

Figure 8. The major game Adults Play: a chart illustration of the concepts of Robert C. Peck (5).

Socializing Versus Sexualizing in Human Relationships

There is some similarity between this category and the first category in that the *whole* of a social relationship becomes more important than just the physical part of a relationship. This is not to say that the physical component of a relationship is unimportant, but rather that the whole relationship increases in significance to the mature adult. It is possible that the wholeness of the relationship can bring more meaning to the physical components. Two persons interacting, who perceive themselves as integrated, self-directed, unique persons are more likely to find deeper meaning to any aspect of a social or sexual relationship than are persons who seek to fill their own feelings of inadequacy through a social or sexual relationship. In such relationships the quality of physical and emotional interaction takes precedence over the quantity of interaction.

A myth about aging is that sex and sexuality decrease in importance in the older person. However, sexual interaction continues to be a valuable part of a relationship for many older people. The security, belonging, and self-esteem that partners experience in a long-term relationship can result in a comfortable, ever-developing process. Often in youth the sexual experience is seen from the male perspective as being the "number of conquests possible," and from the female perspective in relation to the "meaningfulness" of the interaction. It may be that as a man and woman age, men become more interested in meaningfulness, and women become more interested in the physical pleasure that accompanies the emotional joy of the relationship.

Cathectic Flexibility Versus Cathectic Impoverishment

The concept of cathectic flexibility is exemplified by people who are basically secure with who they are as developing, mature adults whose lives are becoming more enriched. They have observed and learned from interaction with others, discovered the beauty of differences, and find less need to be exact and have things divided into discrete categories. They are more able to adjust, to be flexible, and to "give in to" the wishes of others without compromising their own priorities and needs. Such people can be called cathectically flexible.

On the other hand, people who feel somewhat insecure, do not feel as if they belong, and have not developed much self-esteem are very likely to remain inflexible and can be described as cathectically impoverished. They may even become more rigid, because the rigidity provides security that is not available from other sources. This security gives them some sense of belonging and self-esteem.

Extremes of flexibility or inflexibility generally are not indicative of psychological health. For example, if people are so flexible that they always give in to the wishes of others and do not maintain the things in their lives that provide for security, belonging, and self-esteem, they would be wishy-washy, unhappy people, who are very unsure of their own identity. Securities (or inflexibilities) of various kinds are needed to provide some structure and limits for the life of any person. Furthermore, people who are aware of and interested in their own psychological development will periodically examine their priorities in relation to security.

Mental Flexibility Versus Mental Rigidity

Peck's own description of mental flexibility and rigidity bears repeating. He says, "Some people learn to master their experiences, achieve a degree of detached perspective on them, and make use of them as provisional guides to the solution of new issues. There are other people who seem to become dominated by their experiences. They take the patterns of events and actions which they happen to have encountered, as a set of fixed inflexible rules which almost automatically govern their subsequent behavior" (5, p. 90). Thus, willingness to learn, both from self and others, and willingness to change are important to mental growth. As persons age and their experiences increase, questions arise about incongruities in what is observed, heard, and experienced. These questions, which can come from intuition and the creative process within, provide a base for mental flexibility. Mental flexibility may be the basis for more questions than answers, but the openness that accompanies such flexibility provides a fertile bed for growth toward meaningful answers to a person's dilemmas.

Religion can provide an example of both mental flexibility and mental rigidity. Religion provides a certain amount of security and belonging for any person who is even peripherally involved in the religion of his or her choice. The difference between flexibility and rigidity, however, relates to the source of the criteria by which that religion is practiced. For example, people who properly and systematically follow the rituals and guidelines that have been established, and do this with few questions and little doubt, are readily labeled as religious people. These people are often seen as "good" members of the group who help to maintain the institution of religion. Such a person most likely sees faith as being personal yet has difficulty dealing with questions, which others raise, that imply doubt. Furthermore, doubt may be viewed as unacceptable. These people can be described as mentally rigid.

Conversely, people who come to religion with a certain amount of questioning and doubtfulness, can be described as mentally flexible. They may be seen as "problems" to organized religion because of personal doubt. These people examine the tenets of faith and the rituals and guidelines of their religion in relationship to subjective experience with the Supreme Being. These people integrate their theology, their philosophy, and their psychology. When incongruities arise between identity as a person in relation to God and what established religion says, these people deal with the incongruities. To do this, mental flexibility is necessary. It is very possible that the mentally flexible person will find it necessary to reject portions of former beliefs and replace them with those that are more consistent with current subjective experience.

Whether we are speaking of religion, philosophy, or life-style, a certain amount of mental flexibility promotes the examination of ideology so change and growth can take place. It is through this process that a person finds answers, meaning, and a certain amount of congruity in personhood. In Maslow's terms, this process is a component of self-actualization.

Old Age

Ego Differentiation Versus Work-Role Preoccupation

Since older people are living longer, they live beyond the years of what has been societally determined as "work" into the "retirement years." Furthermore, the American way of life is based on the "work ethic," and work roles are valued highly in our society. Therefore, ego differentiation versus work-role preoccupation is an important category to consider. Throughout life, in social interactions, persons are often identified by their role in a job rather than by who they are as persons. Dealing with the question of self-worth or the value of each person as a unique human being versus the value of that person in the work oriented role is a difficult task.

Cultural values of financial status, which accompany the work role factor, compound the issue. Even the current system for providing financial support in retirement is predicated on the person's income while he or she was in the work role.

Because of society's established value system, the self-worth of a person often reflects the values of the surrounding society. There is some overlap of Erikson's and Peck's categories here. Moreover, there may be some male-female differences that relate to whether the woman's primary work-role was as a housewife rather than in an occupation outside the home. Peck states, "For most men, the ability to find a sense of self-worth in activities beyond the 'job' seems to make the most difference between a despairing loss of meaning in life, and a continued, vital interest in living. For many women, this stage may arrive when their 'vocational' role as mother is removed by the departure of the grown children. In that case, this crisis stage might well come in middle age, for many women" (5, p. 90).

However, older people need to value themselves for who they are as persons rather than for who they are as workers if a sense of self-worth is to be achieved. Persons who, in the middle years, dealt with "valuing wisdom versus valuing physical powers" have successfully developed a sense of self-worth through the years and will most likely cope effectively with work-role preoccupation after retirement. These people have found a balance between work and personal identity. On the other hand, people who are "workaholics", people who are always too busy to take vacations during their working years, and those who have difficulty relaxing and "having a good time" may have a great deal of difficulty with the drastic change in role that retirement brings. In other words, the concept of ego differentiation supports the theory that older people should prepare earlier in life for retirement years by having diversified interests and activities.

Body Transcendence Versus Body Preoccupation

This category relates very closely to the second category of middle age in that both focus on a person's body-centered priorities. In addition to the sex-role/sex-activity issue, the older person must often deal with an increase in physical health problems such as arthritis, heart disease, and maturity-onset diabetes mellitus. Often such health problems are chronic rather than acute and can therefore be treated so the person perceives his/herself as basically healthy. However, the person is aware that the health problem exists, and this awareness can be accentuated by physical pain or discomfort and by certain limitations of activity.

Physical "givens" of old age are that there is a decline in resistance to illness and recuperative powers, and an increase in "aches and pains." On the other hand, as a person ages, there is an increase in accumulated knowledge and life experience. This increase is often called wisdom.

The older person who views *self* as "more than physical body" is more likely to be able to endure some discomfort so the things in life which bring meaning and satisfaction can be pursued. For example, the discomfort of arthritis can be submerged by meaningful human relationships or creative mental activity.

The basis for psychological health in relation to body awareness and use is firmer if the person learns to value his or herself as more than a physical body as he or she ages. However, the critical test of these values often comes in old age when the reality of the body's deterioration and decline must be faced.

Ego Transcendence Versus Ego Preoccupation

Another "given" of aging is that someday death will take place. A person's lifelong process of becoming a whole, integrated being is very important to facing the inevitability of death. Mental flexibility, which developed during middle age, is a useful resource in moving from ego preoccupation to transcendence. When Erikson speaks of ego integrity versus despair, he observes that people who are not satisfied with their life accomplishments feel despair and often fear death (6). Another approach to death, passive resignation, can also be seen as a form of ego preoccupation. Passive resignation may be a way of denying that death will occur by not facing its reality. On the other hand, passive resignation may represent a desire to get through the experience quickly, a form of seeking for immediate gratification.

In contrast, people with ego transcendence or ego integrity can be described as having a vital, gratifying absorption in the future. People who have ego integrity are able to look beyond or to transcend self, looking to the happiness and welfare of others. They are interested in making a better world for familial and cultural descendents. They are concerned with a sense of world order, spiritual integrity, and wholeness. Their caring for and love of the human ego is postnarcissistic; and, although they care about themselves, seeking to defend their own dignity and life-style against physical and economic threats, their ultimate concerns are other directed (6). Moreover, they seek to remain physically and emotionally active in their interactions with significant others.

Another "given" of this life period is the loss of significant others. When the grieving process associated with such a loss is experienced with some completeness, people are likely to have less fear of their own death and an attitude of readiness to die coupled with a willingness or eagerness to live as long as life has meaning.

When developmental theories are compared, it is readily evident that much more emphasis is placed on the first half of life. It is true that both physiological and psychological changes occur more rapidly during the first six years of life than at any other time in life (see Fig. 9). In addition, all of a person's basic intellectual operations have usually been developed by adolescence. However, it is possible that adult use of intellectual skills merits study, for there may be some unidentified skills that contribute to the development of what is classified as wisdom or experiental knowledge.

After maturity is achieved, physiological changes are minimal and psychological changes are more gradual and less tied to specific chronological ages. Nevertheless, these changes are important to achievement of ego integrity during the second half of life. The person who has ego integrity readily shares self and insights with others. Erikson suggests that the child learns trust in interaction with an

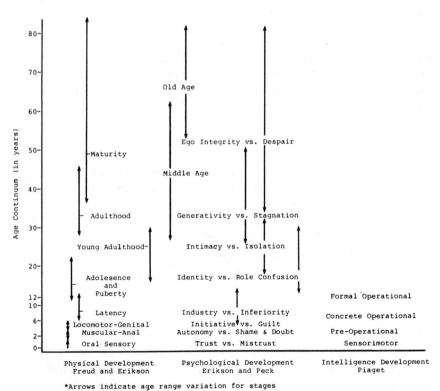

Figure 9. Development throughout life.

adult who displays ego integrity (6). Thus, psychological development comes full circle through meaningful human interaction.

Developmental theories are one approach to describing a person's psychological health, however, theories that focus on motivation for behavior are also helpful in understanding the whole person.

MOTIVATION THEORIES: TOOLS FOR ASSESSMENT OF PSYCHOLOGICAL HEALTH

Needs Motivation

As mentioned previously, Abraham Maslow, one of the founders of humanistic psychology, has devised a hierarchical classification of human motivation based on what he saw as universal human needs (see Table 6) (7). An individual's motivation for behavior throughout life is closely tied to the person he/she becomes and the amount of psychological health he/she experiences.

Maslow divided his hierarchy into two major categories: deficiency needs and metaneeds. Deficiency needs (basic needs) are described as being prepotent, that is, the fundamental physiological needs must be met at a satisfactory level before the intermediate needs of security, belonging and self-esteem can be focused on by a person. Even within the physiological needs there is a hierarchy, which is based on the survival needs of an organism.

When their deficiency needs have been met at a reasonable level, people then are able to focus on growth needs. Growth needs are also classified as self-actualization needs. The term *self-actualization* is described in various ways, however, Maslow described this concept through case studies of persons he believed to be self-actualized. Maslow characterized a self-actualized person as:

· being realistically oriented
· being acceptant of self, others, and the natural world
· being spontaneous
· having an air of detachment
· having a need for privacy
· centering on problems rather than self
· autonomous and independent in relation to culture and environment
· having a nonstereotyped appreciation for people and things
· having profound spiritual experiences, not necessarily religious in nature

· identifying with humankind in general
· being democratic
· having intimate relationships which are deeply emotional, not superficial
· exhibiting moral standards of conduct
· resisting conformity to culture
· having a sense of humor which is philosophical, not hostile
· creative
· transcending, rather than just coping with, the environment (8)

Creativeness is the self-actualization characteristic that is frequently mentioned, however, the other characteristics are equally important if self-actualization is used as a criterion for assessment of psychological health.

In some of his writings, Maslow also pointed out that the person who is functioning at the metaneed level has needs for justice, beauty, goodness, order, and unity.

It is interesting that an analysis of what Erikson described as ego-integrity fits closely with Maslow's description of the self-actualized person.

Locus of Control Construct

Another motivation theory that has been studied extensively in recent years is the locus of control construct, developed by Bernard Weiner (see Fig. 10). Descriptions of persons who have achieved ego-integrity or are self-actualized are quite similar to descriptions of persons who have an internal locus of control. People with an internal locus of control believe in their own ability to accomplish goals that they are motivated to accomplish, and they also believe strongly that whether the task is accomplished or not is primarily because of their own effort to achieve the task. On the other hand, people whose locus of control is primarily external believe that luck has an important role in their success in any task they undertake, and they see success or failure as relating to the difficulty of the task rather than to their own ability (9).

The locus of control construct can be a useful tool in the assessment of client's psychological health. Studies have been done using the locus of control construct to examine people's loss of perceived control.

When persons experience loss of perceived control in one or several incidents in their lives, a pervasive and profound reaction occurs, and they perceive a more generalized loss of control (10). Helplessness, "a perceived inability to effect one's fate meaningfully is the natural re-

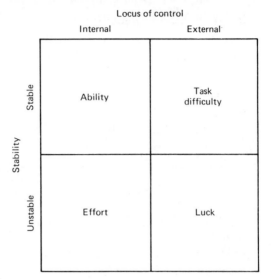

Figure 10. Locus of control construct.

sponse to deprivation and denigration and, in turn, is a source of immature and poor coping behavior" (10).

Thus the construct, locus of control, meshes well with the nursing profession's goal to assist clients in coping with experiences as they perceive them. If clients perceive their experiences as being those over which they have control, the locus of control is from within, or internal. If, on the other hand, they perceive that they do not have control over their experiences, the locus of control is primarily external, and a nursing challenge or problem may exist.

CLIENT PERCEPTIONS

Perception of Self

What is meant by "perception"? Perception in relation to belief about self, personal health status, and life situation has been used several times thus far in this book. Perception is a sensory process that uses the five senses and mental skills to bring meaning to information collected from the environment. Initially, then, perception appears to be a somewhat mechanistic process engaging body and mind synergistically. However, there is more to the process. Often, generalizations are made in response to a current sensation using conscious and unconscious information from past experiences with similar sensations. For example, a person may say "I feel good, therefore, I am healthy."

Information from a person's knowledge base is also used to sort sensory stimuli. Moreover, a perceptual set, a readiness or expectation for how or what a stimulus will be, can influence how a person perceives a sensation. There is often an attitudinal component to a perceptual set. For example, people who believe that wisdom and experience compensate for some of the less desirable physical changes of aging will perceive chronological age progression in a more positive way than will people who believe that getting old is to be dreaded as an incurable disease.

Neugarten, in reviewing the years of study she and her colleagues have done on patterns of aging states, "it has become increasingly evident that each person interprets his present situation in terms of what his expectations have been" (11). She says that expectations often relate to people's perception of their place in time or to an age referent. For example, people might comment on their health status in comparison with that of peers or with the health and longevity of ancestors. If a client's parents died in their 50s, the client may believe that having lived to be 65 is a special accomplishment.

Perception of Time and Its Meaning

In addition to the cultural components of time orientation (see Chap. 2), perception of time and its value changes as people progress through the various developmental stages of life. A cogent outline of time and its meaning is provided by Clements (12). He says that time in youth seems to be limitless and variable and a sense of future time is predominant. During the middle years the finiteness of personal time enters a person's awareness, and the finite future is perceived. During early old age awareness of past time increases, and "early old age is a time for catching up." In old age a sense of "now" surfaces, and the value of time remaining is more precious.

A study by Chiriboga (13) in which subjects were asked, "What do you think is the best age to be?" produced some interesting results. The subjects in this study ranged in age from 16 to 67. Approximately 60% of the subjects said that the teen years and the 20s were the best, 18% of the subjects said the 30s were the best years, and only 8% said the 50s or 60s were the best age. No one selected the 70s or 80s even though these years represented the remaining available time for about one-third of the subjects. The subjects were also asked "What do you think is the worst age to be?" The teen years were the worst according to 45% of the subjects, and over seventy was the worst age to be according to 27%. Interestingly, an age close to a current age was chosen as "best age to be" by younger persons, but only a very small percentage of people in their 50s and 60s chose a proximate age as the "best to be." What these findings say about perception of self and present age is not clear, but the implication exists that "young is better" and that old age is to be dreaded rather than eagerly anticipated.

Another study that looked at subjective speed of time showed that as a person ages the value of time tends to increase (14). How persons perceive their own progression through time and the importance of that progression influences their perception of self. If people in early old age, as defined by Clements, can look back with a sense of satisfaction about their lives up to current time, then they have a positive frame of reference for present and future experience with time.

An interesting component of Clement's presentation relates to his description of old age as being oriented to a sense of "now." "The experience of 'now' is a case of radical freedom in which the aged person is freed from the subjective bondages of time as perceived in the previous ages of life" (12). He goes on to say that this freedom can be seen as either a negative or a positive experience. If this freedom is expressed in denial or "death" of earlier life, then the "nowness" is probably a negative experience. However, if the freedom is seen as a process that prepares persons for their ultimate destiny, then the "now" is a positive, active experience and freedom to grow into the unknown future exists. Clements' ideas about time perception tie in well with both Erikson's concept of ego-integrity and Peck's idea of ego transcendence.

Thus, perception of time and its meaning is important in the clients' perception of self as they consider who they are currently in comparison with their past sense of purpose and being and as they consider what the future holds for them as people in relation to remaining time.

Perception of Intellectual Abilities

Although most of the research on intellectual skills relates to children and young people, more studies on the intellectual abilities of older people are now being done. However, theories that outline the mental and intellectual development of older people, such as Piaget developed for children, (see Fig. 9) are not available.

In a society where change, speed, and youth are valued, wisdom, contemplation, and reminiscence are often not valued. Therefore, old is perceived as negative; and it is assumed that because there is a difference in skills between young and old, the skills of the older person are somehow less valuable, and the intelligence of an older person is therefore decreased. In fact, within the past several decades, some authorities on mental abilities have written that mental decline is to be expected in aging people along with observable decreases in physical stamina and speed.

We would do well at times to read the works of the ancient philosophers. Cicero, writing during the first century BC, said, "old men retain their intellects well enough if only they keep their minds active and fully employed" (15). As far as we know the only research data he used were his own experience and the experience of those he observed and knew. For instance, in his treatise "On Old Age" he reminds us that Plato was at his writing desk when he died at the age of 81. Another acquaintance of his wrote a personal eulogy in his ninety-fourth year, but lived another five years. It seems that the Greek philosophers valued the wisdom, influence, thought, reason, and prudence they found most old people to have. Somehow, in American society, we have moved rather far from this belief; nonetheless, we may now be more accepting of the idea that older people do have intellectual skills, sometimes far beyond the abilities of younger persons.

Even though there are data supporting the notion of continued and increased intellectual ability in older persons, collecting information on their perception of their own mental abilities is important during nursing assessment. Even so, some knowledge of research findings provides the nurse with the background needed to assess a client holistically.

One of the most interesting research findings in the last decade is that data collected on intellectual abilities in longitudinal studies differ considerably from data obtained in cross-sectional studies. According to Schaie and Labouvie, "traditional interpretations of intellectual decrement need to consider more carefully the confounding factor of cultural-historical change. . . . In times of rapid cultural and technological change it is primarily in relation to younger populations that the aged can be described as deficient, and it is erroneous to interpret such cross-sectional age differences as indicating ontogenetic change patterns" (16, p.317).

Much research, including longitudinal studies, supports the idea that the "fluid dimensions of intelligence," that is, things such as speed and fluency abilities, do decrease slightly as a person ages. However, longitudinal studies have indicated that "crystalized dimensions of intelligence," such as verbal meaning, space, and reasoning, do not decline and sometimes increase as a person ages. In fact, some research data demonstrate a slight increase in fluid intelligence when the older person engages in certain activities (16, 17).

Research findings on the mental abilities of older people are encouraging. The question still exists: how can these positive findings influence personal perception of mental abilities of older persons? Some responsibility lies with the health professionals who relate to healthy older persons. Too often the unstated expectations that a health professional has of an older client exert some influence on the client's beliefs and behaviors. Therefore, it is the nurse's responsibility to teach individuals and groups that older people have continued potential and abilities, as well as to assess the client's abilities accurately and objectively.

HETEROGENEITY OF THE AGING POPULATION

Studies that evaluate the physical, mental, and social abilities of the older population have demonstrated equivocal results. The diversity of the research results supports the idea that as persons age they are less likely to conform to conventional and external standards and more likely to become more like themselves and less like their peers. Schaie and Labouvie's findings about the changes in intellectual abilities among older people certainly support the concept of heterogeneity, in that mental ability was found to be increased in some older people and to be decreased in others.

The various findings about active and passive approaches to successful aging (see Fig. 7) also support the idea of heterogeneity. In other words, there is a broad range of life-styles in aging that fall within "normal range." Moreover, people have the right to chose whether they will be "rocking chair" or "jogging" people.

According to Cicero, "old age is respectable just as long as it asserts itself, maintains its proper rights, and is not enslaved by anyone" (15). Such a philosophy about aging increases the freedom that a person has to be "his own person." It seems, too, that the increased value time has for older persons reiterates to them the importance of using the time that remains to achieve personal goals rather than to "blend" with the desires of others in the environment.

Polly Francis says, "Length is only one dimension of life. So I try to avoid an exaggerated concern about my state of health—and I refuse to deny myself some little pleasures I am told are not good for me. If I want to drink a cup of coffee at midnight or go without my rubbers, what of it? A little private rebellion now and then can relieve a harmful tension. I've been indiscreet all my life and I'm still around as I begin my ninety-first year" (18). Writing with a slightly different emphasis two years later, she said, "As my sense of detachment grows and I feel less earthbound, a new kind of freedom, a release settles over me" (19).

Thus, a view of aging as a heterogeneous process provides for a sense of freedom and dignity with diversity of expression and involvement. McLeish gives numerous examples of persons, whom he classifies as Ulyssean adults. These are persons who either launch into totally new careers or creativity during the second half of life or those who remain "richly productive within the sphere of creativity where he or she has long performed." He later points out that these persons are "not oblivious to the judgement of others, but the basis of evaluation lies within. . . ." (20). A certain amount of freedom from external constraints facilitates this personal and creative response to life, which, when compared with "norms" or life-styles of others, results in a population that only can be described as varied, nonsimilar, or heterogeneous.

MISNOMERS OF BEHAVIORAL VARIATIONS

This very heterogeneity, or decrease in "sameness," along with attitudinal biases against the aging process, results in labels or categorizations with negative connotations. The motivation for applying labels to individuals or groups often comes from a lack of knowledge about the behaviors that are being observed or from a fear of either the behavior or the person who is "behaving."

Often behaviors in older people that are similar to behaviors in younger people are labeled or described differently simply because of the client's age. For example, a younger person who is sick physically and is behaving in a withdrawn, depressed manner is described as assuming the sick role, whereas an older person who may be experiencing a loss or illness and behaves in a depressed manner is described as being disengaged or becoming senile. *Senility* is a term that in current usage is meaningless because it has many meanings and is, therefore, not descriptive; it is merely a pejorative term. A young person who behaves in unconventional ways or who expresses hostility or cynicism is labeled as adventuresome, unique, or a nonconformist, whereas the older person may be called eccentric or may be labeled as senile. Polly Francis observed that "senility is a convenient peg upon which to hang our nonconformity" (18).

Another example of misnomers in relation to behavior is that when a young person fails to remember something, it is ascribed to the fact that he is very busy and therefore cannot recall the information at the moment, or he is concentrating and cannot think about the new topic. The older person, on the other hand, is often labeled as forgetful, or as losing his memory; and it is presumed both by the person who cannot remember, and by the observers, that there is no hope for memory loss in the elderly.

Therefore, it is assumed that memory loss is to be expected in old age. This assumption is not based on fact, but on a long-standing perpetuation of a myth. Memory loss of any significance occurs as a symptom of a pathological process and is not a normal part of aging. Circulatory problems are probably the most common cause of pathological memory loss.

A certain amount of normal forgetting occurs with length of life. The human brain has some limitations in the amount of conscious information that is readily available for recall. People of any age who are focusing in depth on a thought pattern or content area can have temporary memory loss for other content areas not of current interest or importance to them. However, when information that is stored in the memory is needed, a recall process is activated to facilitate surfacing of the information. This is usually a process of association of easy to recall information with difficult to recall information. The phrase "cast my mind back," used often by the characters in Agatha Christie mysteries, refers to this memory recall process. Older people who assume that it is normal for old people to lose their memory may not exercise their recall processes and thus create a self-fulfilling prophecy when temporary memory loss exists. This is unfortunate, since the recall methods that worked for persons throughout the years are the same methods that will work for them in old age.

It can be theorized that, as priorities change with aging and a person becomes more transcendent in life-style, some information is of little importance and, therefore, is not remembered. Memory, however, is an important resource for the older person, as Butler and Lewis point out when speaking of life review or reminiscence (21).

PSYCHOLOGICAL RESOURCES OF THE AGED: A SUMMARY

Resources that older people have to cope successfully with the challenges and losses they experience include the wisdom that comes from a lifetime of effective coping, the process of reminiscence, religion, and their realistic perspective of time. Effective movement through the developmental crises and challenges during the first half of life, as well as during middle age, provides a variety of effective approaches to new challenges and experiences.

Butler sees reminiscence in the aged as a natural, "universal mental process characterized by the progressive return to consciousness of past experiences . . ." (22). It provides the person with an opportunity to work through previously unresolved conflicts and to review and to reintegrate happy and sad experiences of the past. The process of reminiscence can bring a new wholeness to persons and can add to their wisdom, as well as improve their time perspective.

Religion is an important psychological resource, especially for the person who has internalized a belief system and achieved a mentally flexible but active faith.

In essence, the persons who people have become is their greatest psychological resource. If people have progressed successfully through the adult developmental stages, they can use their maturational experience to cope effectively with new ambiguities, challenges, and losses.

REFERENCES

1. Neugarten BL, Havighurst RJ, Tobin SS: The Measurement of Life Satisfaction. *J Gerontol* 16:134–143, 1961.
2. Havighurst RJ: Personality and Patterns of Aging. *Gerontologist* 8:20–23, 1968.
3. Neugarten BL, Havighurst RJ, Tobin SS: Personality and patterns of aging, in Neugarten BL (ed): *Middle Age and Aging.* Chicago, The University of Chicago Press, 1968.
4. Kimmel DC: *Adulthood and Aging.* New York, John Wiley and Sons, 1974, p 18.
5. Peck RC: Psychological developments in the second half of life, in Neugarten BL (ed): *Middle Age and Aging.* Chicago, The University of Chicago Press, 1968, pp. 88–92.

6. Erikson EH: *Childhood and Society*, ed 2. New York, WW Norton and Company, 1963.
7. Maslow AH: *Motivation and Personality*. New York, Harper & Row, 1954.
8. Maslow AH: *Toward a Psychology of Being*. New York, D Van Nostrand Company, 1962.
9. Weiner B: *Theories of Motivation: From Mechanisms to Cognition*. Chicago, Markham, 1972.
10. Lefcourt HM: *Locus of Control: Current Trends in Theory and Research*. New York, John Wiley and Sons, 1976.
11. Neugarten BL: Personality and the aging process. *Gerontologist* 12:12, 1972.
12. Clements WM: Thoughts on a theology of aging: time and meaning in the second half of life. Paper presented at the University of Iowa, November, 1978.
13. Chiriboga DA: Evaluated time: a life course perspective. *J Gerontol* 33:388–393, 1978.
14. Wallach MA, Green LR: On age and the subjective speed of time, in Neugarten BL (ed): *Middle Age and Aging*. Chicago: The University of Chicago Press, 1968.
15. Cicero MT: On Old Age. In *Gateway to the Great Books*, Vol 10. Chicago, Encyclopedia Britannica, 1963.
16. Schaie KW, Labouvie-Vief G: Generational versus ontogenetic components of change in adult cognitive behavior: a fourteen-year cross-sequential study. *Develop Psychol* 10:305–320, 1974.
17. Plemons JK, Willis SL, Baltes PB: Modifiability of fluid intelligence in aging: a short-term longitudinal training approach. *J Gerontol* 33:224–231, 1978.
18. Francis, P. The autumn of my life, in *The Washington Post*, March 16, 1975.
19. Francis, P: Awakening. *Perspective on Aging* 6:24–25, 1977.
20. McLeish JAB: *The Ulyssean Adult-Creativity in the Middle and Later Years*. Toronto, McGraw-Hill Ryerson, 1976.
21. Butler RN, Lewis MI: *Aging and Mental Health*. St. Louis, CV Mosby Company, 1973.
22. Butler RN: *Why Survive? Being Old in America*. New York, Harper & Row, 1975.

ANNOTATED BIBLIOGRAPHY

Birren JE, Schaie KW (eds): *Handbook of the Psychology of Aging*. New York, Van Nostrand Reinhold Company, 1977.

An authoritative reference that provides scientific and professional literature covering a broad range of topics. Biological aspects of behavior, environmental influences and cross-cultural perspectives are among the issues discussed.

Clements WM: *Care and Counselling of the Aging*. Philadelphia, Fortress Press, 1979.

A practical aid written with clergy as the primary audience, but useful to other helping professionals working with elderly clients. Time perspective and some of the developmental crises of aging are discussed.

Hulicka IM: *Empirical Studies in the Psychology and Sociology of Aging*. New York, Thomas Y. Crowell Company, 1977.

A book of abstracts of research literature covering a wide range of psychosocial topics including intellectual functioning, memory, life satisfaction, personality attributes, retirement, passage of time and death. Focus is on aging, not only the aged, so there are abstracts of research on psychological and sociological components of the aging process.

Jarvik LF, Eisdorfer C, Blum, JE: *Intellectual Functioning in Adults*. New York, Springer Publishing Company, 1973.

Clinically applicable research on intellectual capacities of older persons is reported. The value of the developmental psychology of older persons is discussed.

Neugarten BL (ed): *Middle Age and Aging: A Reader in Social Psychology*. Chicago: The University of Chicago Press, 1968.

A useful collection of essays and research reports which covers a broad range of aging issues. Roles, life cycle psychology, psychosocial aging theories, psychosocial health and work and family components of aging are discussed.

chapter five
economic resources
for the aged

The test of our progress is not whether we add more to the abundance of those who have much; it is whether we provide enough for those who have too little.

Franklin D. Roosevelt
Second Inaugural Address, 1937

OUTLINE

The system of chapter divisions (categories) seems somewhat arbitrary when holism is the goal. For example, a cultural perspective looks at the person interacting with all aspects of his culture—belief systems, economics, social networks, and so on. In addition, a discussion of economic resources cannot be totally separated from the social network or from the beliefs held by individuals and groups.

Yet, in urbanized and industrialized America, the major portion of a person's economic resources has moved from the jurisdiction of the family or kinship system to the governmental/political domain. The wage earner is almost automatically plugged into the national economic structure. The fact that every citizen has a social security number ties him into the federal tax system, the social security system, and other nonmonetary benefits of employment.

So the economic resources of retired people are inevitably tied to the economic/political/governmental structure of the larger American society. This chapter will examine the economic resources that are intertwined with this governmental structure; Chapter 6 will discuss the kinship component of the economic system, which was introduced in Chapter 2.

On the journey from birth to death, there is a series of events that have significant impact on the life of the person in his or her social environment. Retirement is one of these events, in that a great many changes are triggered. The realistic situation in American society today is that each person's economic resources are tied to the governmental resources and need to be discussed in that context.

Although the nurse is not primarily responsible for assisting a client in obtaining available economic resources, he or she can assess client needs more completely and make appropriate referrals if she or he has some basic knowledge of the resources available. Awareness of the client's experiences may help the nurse to understand the person's reactions to various situations.

Independence and self-reliance are highly valued personal characteristics for most Americans. Therefore, clients are often hesitant to discuss financial status, especially when needs exist. Moreover, nurses may be hesitant, often rightly so, to pursue the topic of finances with clients who demonstrate an unwillingness to discuss the topic. Clients have the right not to share information that they do not desire to share, for whatever reason. Nonetheless, the nurse's responsibility is to be sensitive to potential needs, and whenever appropriate, to share information about available resources with clients. One way of providing information without requiring clients to share more than they wish to share would be to put a simple poster that states where and how to obtain information about Social Security in a clinic area.

Some general and specific information about income, health care, and housing options for the retired, elderly client follows.

BRIEF HISTORY OF RETIREMENT IN AMERICA

For employees, retirement is likely to occur at a preset and predetermined time based on reaching retirement age, which is determined by someone else. In our industrial society, this age has tended to be 65 for most workers. This age was set as the minimum age for retirement in the Social Security Act of 1935, and as is often true, came to be both the minimum and the usual. For other people, however, this "magic age" may have little or no impact of change. For example, the housewife usually continues her regular activities to a much later age. On the other hand, she may have significantly modified her own schedule and activities at age 45 or 55 after the children left home. People who own businesses or who are self-employed may choose either to continue regular activities to a later age than 65 or to retire at an earlier age. These decisions may be related to health conditions, business considerations, or personal interests and are not specifically age related.

There is some trend toward a flexible period for the decision to retire. For some time, the social security program has permitted retirement at age 62 at a somewhat lower benefit level. Private retirement plans often have various income levels dependent on the number of years employed or on some combination of length of employment and age. Professional and self-employed persons may choose to reduce their workload and income over a period of time, on a planned basis, rather than to shift at a given date from working to being retired. Other people will retire from employment, begin drawing their retirement income, and then find other employment, perhaps part time, to occupy time and to provide income.

As the role of a retired person has become more clearly established and acceptable in our society, people find various ways to move in that role, which enable them to make needed adjustments with minimal disruption.

During the early years of the settling and developing of our country, the economy was largely rural in nature. The rural setting was either agricultural or small community and was family and neighborhood based. In this simpler socioeconomic system, families supplied most of their own economic needs, and usually all members of the family were important to the maintenance of the family economy. The extra hands of children and the older members of the household were all important to the unit's economic sufficiency. In this socioeconomic setting, grandpa or grandma were welcome and important members for their productivity, experience, wisdom, and companionship. Their economic security was based in the family, and their physical and social needs were assured by the family unit. For the vast majority of Americans, family structure changed as the United States moved to an industrial economy. Larger cities became the more common place of residence, so the wage earner would be close to the work place. Homes often were smaller than the typical farm house, so there was no longer room for the members of the older generation to live near children and grandchildren.

Opportunities for better salaries, advancement in responsibility, and the necessity of going where specific skills are needed—all parts of an industrial economy—have resulted in greater mobility of workers and their families. Often this means there is great distance between parents and their adult children and between other members of the family.

The change to an urban, industrial economy resulted in meeting needs for food, clothing, and other necessities by exchanging money rather than products; these needs were no longer met within the family. In the industrial socioeconomic system, the family is dependent on wages from the place(s) of employment. We recognize that the industrial economy has made a high standard of living possible for most people in the United States; however, it is also the source of economic problems and insecurity for many people. The economic depressions of the nineteenth century and, more especially, the great depression of the 1930s emphasized that, in this economy, many persons would not be able to develop sufficient resources to take care of their older years.

As early as the 1870s, the industrialized countries of western Europe found that loss of earnings due to accidents, illness, and old age were common to much of the population, and that it was necessary to develop social policies and programs through the government to insure workers against the loss of income that results from these hazards. It was important to the economy to find a means by which people could be insured against the loss of income, that is, have an income to replace the lost earnings, so as to continue to be able to purchase the necessities in a money economy.

The late nineteenth and early twentieth century saw the beginnings of this same social awakening in the United States to the needs of people whose labor was essential to the industrial economy. A few leaders discussed measures to deal with these problems, and state and local governments took actions toward improving working hours and decreasing hazards of injury while working. It was the overwhelming economic crisis of the depression of the 1930s that forced the country into a rapid development of income maintenance measures, through social insurance and public assistance. These new programs were accomplished through the enactment by Congress of the Social Security Act in August 1935. This act encompassed many programs to respond to the loss of income, including programs for people who were unemployed, old, disabled, blind, or in a home without a wage earner (dependent children). Of special interest to us, however, is the retirement program established as an insurance program entitled Old Age Insurance and a second program entitled Old Age Assistance, which were jointly funded by federal and state governments and administered by states.

The enactment of this pioneering legislation established the concept of retirement as an appropriate role in our society and provided some income security for the older citizen. Since 1935, changes have been made to provide for other problems. Of great significance to the older population was the addition in 1965 of Title XVIII, an amendment to the Social Security Act, to provide an insurance program to meet part of the costs of medical and hospital bills for retired persons past age 65. Also, in 1965 another amendment, creating Title XIX to the Social Security Act, established a program called Medicaid to assist elderly persons receiving Old Age Assistance to pay costs of medical and hospital care (Medicaid is also available to younger persons who qualify.).

In 1972, another major change in the Social Security Act established the Supplemental Security Income (S.S.I.) program. Through this legislation the program of Old Age Assistance in the original act changed from plans that varied from state to state to a basic program administered by the federal government through the Social Security Administration.

The depression years also increased governmental awareness that many people did not have adequate housing, and some programs for public housing were developed as early as 1937. By 1956, Americans had become more aware that older persons had special housing needs and recognized that adequate housing was priced out of the reach of many people because of reduced income at retirement. Since that time various policies and programs have been instituted to improve housing for the older population.

Throughout the twentieth century, as America has become an industrialized, urbanized economy and society, the number of people over age 65 has increased notably (see Table 1 in chap. 1). Improved general health, better medical and health services, and a higher standard of living have contributed to this great increase in the older population. In the past 30 years our society has become increasingly concerned that all older people have a "decent" standard of living during their later years. Society has also become aware that significant numbers of older people do not have resources to provide for themselves at that level and that special needs create problems for the older person.

Governmental response to this concern resulted in the White House Conference on Aging in 1961 and 1971. These conferences have stimulated states and local communities to study the needs and problems of their older population to assess services available and needs for new services. The White House Conference structure has brought national attention to these needs and has encouraged the development of national and state social policy through legislation to assure meeting the needs of our older people.

The concept of comprehensive public policy on the elderly population in the United States is well stated in the Older Americans Act of July 14, 1965. (Public Law 89−73). These broad statements of public policy provide a framework for further analysis of problems and for developing and funding services for the elderly. They also serve to provide a perspective for our society.

TITLE I—DECLARATION OF OBJECTIVES: DEFINITIONS

Declaration of Objectives for Older Americans

Sec. 101. The Congress hereby finds and declares that, in keeping with the traditional American concept of the inherent dignity of the individual in our democratic society, the older people of our Nation are entitled to, and it is the joint and several duty and responsibility of the governments of the United States and their political subdivisions to assist our older people to secure equal opportunity to the full and free enjoyment of the following objectives:

(1) An adequate income in retirement in accordance with the American standard of living.

(2) The best possible physical and mental health which science can make available and without regard to economic status.

(3) Suitable housing, independently selected, designed and located with reference to special needs and available at costs which older citizens can afford.

(4) Full restorative services for those who require institutional care.
(5) Opportunity for employment with no discriminatory personnel practices because of age.
(6) Retirement in health, honor, dignity—after years of contribution to the economy.
(7) Pursuit of meaningful activity within the widest range of civic, cultural, and recreational opportunities.
(8) Efficient community services which provide social assistance in a coordinated manner and which are readily available when needed.
(9) Immediate benefit from proven research and knowledge which can sustain and improve health and happiness.
(10) Freedom, independence, and the free exercise of individual initiative in planning and managing their own lives (1).

Within the framework of these broad goals for all elderly citizens, a system of social policies and programs is being created to enable the retiree to make the changes that accompany the transition to retirement. Usually there is a reduction in income. Upon retirement there may be increased costs in hospital and doctors' services, and it may be desirable to make different living arrangements. Public programs offer help to maintain income on loss of wages, help pay hospital and doctors' bills, and a variety of housing choices for the elderly. Despite the availability of these programs, the nurse will occasionally find, among the people served, a number of people who do not qualify for any benefits even though they may have very real needs. The person may not have been employed long enough to qualify for a social security or private business retirement benefit, or he or she may have sufficient assets, as defined by social security legislation, (e.g., a house) and may not be eligible to receive S.S.I. but may still have insufficient income to purchase the necessities of life. This is to say that the system of programs to aid the retired, elderly person still has gaps, and some people may be in great need because they do not fulfill the requirements of the programs available.

The newly defined status of "retiree" has stimulated the development of courses or workshops designed to help the middle-aged person to learn about that phase of life, it's possibilities, and problems and to plan realistically. Such services are now provided by some companies for their employees or by colleges, community colleges, and adult education programs. To make use of any of these programs the person must learn about them and determine what will best meet his or her needs.

In the remainder of this chapter societal policies and programs designed to enable people to make the changes associated with assuming the role of retiree will be identified and discussed briefly. These programs cover three major areas: *1)* income maintenance, or substitute income, *2)* hospital and medical care costs, and *3)* housing.

INCOME MAINTENANCE PROGRAMS

Social Security Retirement Benefits

As people begin to plan for retirement, they become aware that their salary will cease; they therefore begin to look for substitute income, such as that derived from social security benefits, railroad retirement benefits and retirement benefits provided by employer, unions, or insurance. Most Americans are eligible for the benefits of the social security program known as Old Age Insurance initiated by the passage of the Social Security Act in August 1935. By the late 1970s, more than 90% of the work force in the United States has been covered by the provisions of this social insurance program. Each employed person is aware of this program since each paycheck shows the amount that has been deducted and paid into social security trust funds (from which the monthly retirement check will be paid).

Eligibility requirements for social security benefits state that a person needs to have been employed in a job that is covered under the insurance program for at least 40 quarters (10 years). The amount of the retirement check is determined by a formula based on the average earnings and length of employment, and eligibility is contingent on leaving the work force. The usual age for eligibility for full benefits is 65, but a person may retire at 62 with a reduced benefit.

The formula for determining the amount of benefit is skewed somewhat to aid people who have had lower average earnings in an attempt to assure some reasonable level of income for all people. Table 7 shows the level of social security retirement income as related to various levels of average earnings. In addition to the benefit available to a retiree, a benefit is also available to the dependent spouse and for children under age 18 or 22, if in school.

As a result of continuing inflation in the economy, the Social Security Act now provides for a cost of living adjustment once each year to compensate to some extent for increasing costs.

In July 1978, 20,981,239 retired workers and their spouses were receiving retirement benefits totaling $5,086,842,000 (2). The average benefit for the retired worker for this same month was $277.86 and for

Table 7. Social Security Retirement Benefits.

Monthly retirement benefits (payable starting July 1978)

Average yearly earnings	For Workers Retirement at 65	at 64	at 63	at 62	For Dependents[1] Spouse at 65 or child	at 64	at 63	at 62	Family[2] benefits
$923 or less	121.80	113.70	105.60	97.50	60.90	55.90	50.80	45.70	182.70
1,200	156.70	146.30	135.90	125.40	78.40	71.90	65.40	58.80	235.10
2,600	230.10	214.80	199.50	184.10	115.10	105.50	95.90	86.40	345.20
3,000	251.80	235.10	218.30	201.50	125.90	115.40	104.90	94.50	384.90
3,400	270.00	252.00	234.00	216.00	135.00	123.80	112.50	101.30	434.90
4,000	296.20	276.50	256.80	237.00	148.10	135.70	123.40	111.10	506.20
4,400	317.30	296.20	275.00	253.90	158.70	145.40	132.20	119.10	562.50
4,800	336.00	313.60	291.20	268.80	168.00	153.90	140.00	126.00	612.70
5,200	353.20	329.70	306.20	282.60	176.60	161.80	147.20	132.50	662.70
5,600	370.60	345.90	321.20	296.50	185.30	169.80	154.40	139.00	687.10
6,000	388.20	362.40	336.50	310.60	194.10	177.80	161.70	145.60	712.10
6,400	405.60	378.60	351.60	324.50	202.80	185.80	169.00	152.10	737.10
6,800	424.10	395.90	367.60	339.30	212.10	194.30	176.70	159.10	762.30
7,200	446.00	416.30	386.60	356.80	223.00	204.30	185.80	167.30	788.90
7,600	465.60	434.60	403.60	372.50	232.80	213.30	194.00	174.60	814.70
8,000	482.60	450.50	418.30	386.10	241.30	221.10	201.10	181.00	844.50
8,400	492.90	460.10	427.20	394.40	246.50	225.80	205.40	184.90	862.60
8,800	505.10	471.50	437.80	404.10	252.60	231.40	210.50	189.50	883.80
9,200	516.00	481.60	447.20	412.80	258.00	236.40	215.00	193.50	903.00
9,400	520.40	485.80	451.10	416.40	260.20	238.40	216.80	195.20	910.40
9,600	524.60	489.70	454.70	419.70	262.30	240.30	218.50	196.80	918.00
9,800	530.40	495.10	459.70	424.40	265.20	243.00	221.00	198.90	928.00
10,000	534.70	499.10	463.50	427.80	267.40	245.00	222.80	200.60	935.70

[1] If a person is eligible for both a worker's benefit and a spouse's benefit, the check actually payable is limited to the larger of the two

[2] The maximum amount payable to a family is generally reached when a worker and two family members are eligible.

dependent spouses, $131.17 (3). These benefits are administered by the Social Security Administration of the United States Department of Health, Education and Welfare through district offices located in larger communities. The telephone directory usually lists the nearest office; also, the post office has informational pamphlets describing the social insurance program and listing the location of the nearest office. People wishing to inquire about the retirement program may go to the nearest office, or, if unable to go to the office, they may request that a staff member make a visit to the home. People inquiring about benefits will need their social security number and birth certificate or some other evidence of date of birth. The staff will be able to help determine probable benefits, depending on the planned date of retirement, and will accept applications if the person is ready for such action.

Supplemental Security Income for the Elderly

Old Age Assistance was part of the original Social Security Act and was administered and financed by the federal, state, and local governments. State and local governments operated these programs within guidelines established by the federal government. However, there was great variation in amount of grant, qualifications for eligibility, and manner of administration of the program from one state to another. This variation has been solved for the most part since the 1972 amendments to the Social Security Act made this basically a federally financed and directed program, administered through the Social Security Administration.

Eligibility is determined by each person's financial need rather than by work history and wage levels. Some people, on reaching retirement age, will have little or no savings, and income from social security may be insufficient for living expenses. This program helps people who are ineligible for social security benefits and may be used to supplement social security income and/or other resources to meet their needs. To be eligible for this program, the older person needs to complete an application form and to show what financial resources are available from all sources, including individual savings, insurance, and property. The staff of the Social Security Administration follows established guidelines in assisting an applicant to determine eligibility for a cash benefit to supplement their other resources.

For July 1978, 2,011,438 persons past age 65 received $206,202,000 in federal S.S.I. funds toward meeting their financial needs (3). People aged 65 and over are eligible for benefits if their income and assets are below specified limits. The following information is included to provide understanding of the program and its impact on people. For determining eligibility, the upper limits on other income are $503.40 a quarter for an individual and $755.40 a quarter for a couple (however, in computing income, $60 per quarter from any kind of income is not counted.). In addition, $195.00 of earned income is disregarded. Above that amount, $1 in benefits is deducted for each $2 of earned income. There is also an asset limit of $1,500 for an individual and $2,259 for a couple. Not included in this asset limit is a home, an automobile worth less than $1,200, household goods and personal effects worth less than

$1,500, or life insurance policies having a face value of less than $1,500. The basic federal benefit to an individual is a monthly cash payment of $177.80 ($266.70 for a couple), as of May 1977. This benefit is reduced by $1 for each $1 of unearned income over $20 per month and for each $2 of earned income over $65 (or over $85 if there is no unearned income).

Information about and application forms for this income supplement program, may be obtained through the nearest Social Security office. General information about the program and the location of the nearest Social Security office can be obtained at the local post office or at the offices of the state department of social service or Department of Job Services.

HEALTH CARE COSTS PROGRAMS

Another financial concern of retired persons is medical and hospital care costs and how they will be met. To help meet these costs there are both public programs and private insurance policies. On retirement many people make use of the public programs and also purchase some private insurance to supplement the public insurance coverage. The Social Security Act provides two programs to help meet such costs, Medicare and Medicaid.

Medicare, a social insurance program designed to meet part of the costs of hospital and medical care, was created by the Congress in 1965 through enactment of legislation to add Title XVIII to the Social Security Act. It is composed of two programs: hospital insurance and supplemental medical insurance. Hospital insurance is financed through a payroll tax levied on employees and employers. The supplemental medical insurance program is financed by beneficiary premiums ($7.20 per month in 1978), and federal general tax income. The programs are administered by the Social Security Administration, of the Department of Health, Education and Welfare. Certification of health care providers is contracted to state health agencies as is the payment of claims to intermediaries such as Blue Cross plans and private insurance companies.

To qualify for hospital insurance, a person must be age 65 or over and must be entitled to social security or railroad retirement benefits. Supplemental medical insurance is available to these same people, but they must enroll in the program and pay a monthly premium. Benefits are usually in the form of payments to third parties, that is, hospitals or physicians, for expenses covered under Medicare. Unfortunately, Medicare pays only part of the costs of hospital and medical care, a pattern consistent with private insurance coverage. In January 1978, nearly 21,000,000 retired workers and their spouses were receiving retirement benefits and were eligible for coverage of Medicare. For the period January–February 1978, 1,683,000 bills for payment for hospital care were approved for a total of $2,207,934,000 (4).

Information about this program may be obtained from the Social Security Administration office in your area.

Medicaid is a benefit program provided through Title XIX, another 1965 amendment to the Social Security Act. It is a joint federal-state program. Each state makes its own decision whether to provide this benefit to its citizens, and as of 1978, Arizona is the only state that does not participate. The program is funded by the federal and state governments and administered by state and local governments.

For the person age 65 or over, whose income is limited to the extent that she or he may be eligible for Supplementary Security Income, the Medicaid program helps to meet the cost of hospital and physician care. People whose income and assets are near the margin below which they would be eligible may also qualify for the Medicaid benefits, even though they do not qualify for the S.S.I. payment. This program is a significant benefit to many older people with very limited resources, especially those who need extensive nursing home care. (See the previous section on S.S.I. for general information on determining eligibility.)

Information about this program may be obtained from the state or local public welfare office, which can be located through the telephone book or through inquiry at the courthouse or the post office.

HOUSING

Housing is another area in which the retiree may experience change for various reasons. Some people will plan to stay in their home or apartment and use their leisure time for visiting friends or relatives, for traveling, for gardening, and for a range of other activities that now become possible. For these people, housing is provided and is part of their plan. If, on the other hand, it is desirable to relocate to be near children, grandchildren, or other family; to find a different climate; or to pursue a special interest, there will be a number of choices to consider.

Many people on retiring will have adequate income and resources to purchase another home or condominium or to rent suitable housing. People making such a significant change will often plan several years ahead. Such advance planning provides opportunity to explore various possibilities, both in the type of housing and in geographic locations. Persons with limited financial retirement means may also wish to relocate to different housing. In some communities, special housing for the elderly and retired persons is available. It is becoming more common for housing to be constructed to meet special needs of the older population. On reaching retirement age, some people, even with reduced income, may qualify for some of these special housing provisions, which may afford better housing than they could manage when living on low earnings.

Some of the choices open to and having special appeal to persons at the point of retirement include:

Retirement Villages. Many of these developments are built by private contractors and provide individual dwellings or garden apartments. Residents usually purchase their own units and pay a monthly service charge for maintenance and the use of common facilities. There is an emphasis on recreational facilities, which appeals to the "young old" or middle aged who have retired early, have above average retirement incomes, and look on retirement as a time for relaxation and recreation.

There are other retirement communities with few amenities and minimal community facilities. Their main attraction is the availability of small, low cost homes, often in warm climates.

Mobile home parks are a version of this type of development and may be more or less populated by retired persons. Many do include people of various ages and socioeconomic backgrounds, thus providing an interesting variety of persons in the community.

Apartments and Condominiums. These options of interest to retirees may be built by nonprofit organizations to serve their members and/or by profit-making corporations to provide a desirable living arrangement for people who either can afford to pay a substantial amount of rent or may have funds from the sale of a home to invest in a condominium. Such facilities are likely to have communal areas to provide opportunity for recreational and educational activities.

Retirement Homes. Retirement homes were developed during the 1960s primarily for middle-class people who wished to be free of the responsibilities of a home (mowing grass, gardening, shoveling snow) and to be able to "just lock the door" and travel to visit family or to enjoy new places. These homes usually required the purchase of the apartment and an agreement that on death of the person the apartment belonged to the cooperation. Many of these homes assured the person of lifetime care and had a "health center" (nursing care facility) as part of its services.

This list is but a sampling of the choices of living arrangements available for people to consider on retirement. There are other choices and part of planning for retirement living is to explore resources in the home community or in other communities of interest.

Adequate and suitable housing has been a public concern in our country since legislation about it was passed in 1937. Since the Housing Act of 1959, specific provision has been made for housing for the older population. The Older Americans Act of 1965 included a goal of housing which states, ... "suitable housing, independently selected, designed and located with reference to special needs and available at costs which older citizens can afford."

The Housing Act of 1959, Section 202, made specific provision that nonprofit sponsors could obtain low-interest federal loans for housing for elderly people, either through new construction or through renovation of existing buildings. The Housing and Community Development Act of 1977 (Public Law 95–128) continued and modified this program and provided funding for rental assistance, subsidies for low income persons, and other programs to stimulate the development of housing appropriate to the needs of the elderly.

In response to federal and state legislation focusing on the needs of housing by retired and elderly populations, a number of patterns have developed. Some communities have created public housing commissions or public housing authorities to build and to operate housing especially to meet the needs of the elderly. Recent literature describes several community programs that provide a range of options to respond to the great variety of needs. One such program is under the auspices of the Public Housing Authority of Dade County, Florida, which has a variety of housing and special programs geared to the needs of the elderly population. A report by the Public Housing Authority states:

> Thirty of the sixty public housing sites provide decent housing at low cost for elderly people who cannot remain in their own homes. At 25 sites, the buildings are designed and reserved exclusively for the elderly. In four housing complexes built in the late 1930's and early 1940's, the elderly live side-by-side with younger families. In a new "congregate housing" facility, the elderly who are mobile, but need assistance with dressing, bathing, and housekeeping are provided private apartments, three meals a day in a central dining room, housekeeping services, and assistance in bathing, etc. (5, p.3).

The Public Housing Authority also provides for rental subsidies for low income elderly, as well as assisting owners in rehabilitating housing in which they live (5).

Many communities now have various kinds of housing available for the elderly, some built by private developers and some by nonprofit corporations or by public housing authorities. However, there are often more people eligible for and interested in these facilities than there is space available. Housing for the elderly will often have special facilities such as community rooms for socialization activities, space for clinics or health services, recreational services, and offices for services important to and used by the elderly.

Information about housing for the elderly, and special services that may be available can be obtained from the local Council on Aging, public housing authority, city or county housing office or the local public welfare office.

SUMMARY

This chapter has focused on the public social programs available to elderly citizens to assist in making the financial life style change associated with retirement. It also has identified some of the major political, economic, and social changes during this century that led to the establishment of the role of retired person as acceptable in our society.

Major public policy developments took place in 1935 with the passage of the Social Security Act, which made provision for retirement income through a social insurance program covering the employed workers and through a public assistance program for those not covered or not adequately covered by the social insurance. Amendments to the Social Security Act in 1965 provided Medicare and Medicaid programs to help persons past age 65 to meet the cost of hospital and physician care and some other health costs.

Legislation in 1937 recognized the need for public social policy to assist in the provision of housing for the elderly, and recent changes have instituted new patterns to assist the elderly in achieving adequate housing in neighborhoods of their choice.

The White House Conferences on Aging in 1961 and 1971 have focused on the special needs of the older population and have resulted in public policy goal statements that have guided further developments at national, state, and local levels.

Nurses and social workers often are serving many of the same clients at the same time in trying to meet the multiple needs of people. These two helping professions should work closely together in assessing economic needs and in providing clients with information about available resources.

People in need of economic resource often have established a trusting relationship with a helping professional, and it is usually this person with whom they will discuss economic needs and concerns. The nurse is sometimes this "most trusted" person, therefore, knowledge about available resources, or sources of information about resources, may make the nurse's task easier and service to each person and to the community more effective.

REFERENCES

1. *Older Americans Act of 1965,* Public Law 89–73.
2. *Social Security Bulletin,* Vol 41, No. 11. US Government Printing Office, November 1978, Table M 10, p 36.
3. *Social Security Bulletin,* Vol 41, No. 11. US Government Printing Office, November 1978, Table M 13, p. 39 and 43.
4. *Developments in Aging: 1977.* A Report of the Special Committee on Aging of the United States Senate, Part I. p. 106, US Government Printing Office, 1978, p. 106.
5. Jones P, Rott E, Murphy MB: *A Report on Services to the Elderly 2 Housing: Dade County's Programs to House the Elderly.* Washington, DC, Aging Program, National Association of Counties Research Foundation, 1976.

ANNOTATED BIBLIOGRAPHY

Atchley C: *The Social Forces in Later Life,* ed 2. Belmont, Calif, Wadsworth Publishing Co, 1977.
    The author draws from a wide range of resources to bring together a good basic view of the process of aging in the United States. Material focusing on the person and on some of the impacts of the aging process, as well as on the impact of society on this process serves as a useful base in developing knowledge and understanding of older persons. Particularly helpful is the discussion of the role of retirement in our social structure.
Developments in Aging: 1977. A Report of the Special Committee on Aging of the United States Senate. US Government Printing Office, 1978.

Part 1 provides a summary of the many developments in governmental services that are of special interest to meeting the special needs of the older population. Part 2 includes statistical data and other supplemental material that are helpful in understanding the extent of involvement of the many departments of government.

Gelwicks LE, Newcomer RJ: *Planning Housing Environments for the Elderly.* Washington, DC, National Council on Aging, 1974.

An architect and planner with the aid of an advisory committee have brought together excellent basic data and viewpoints to emphasize the importance to this special population of good housing and good services to meet the varied and changing needs of this increasing segment of population. Underlying philosophy is made real in specific recommendations for planning and constructing desirable housing.

Turner JB (ed): *Encyclopedia of Social Work.* Washington DC, National Association of Social Workers, 1977.

Special articles on aging, housing, retirement, and social insurance are useful in providing an overview of the particular topic; a brief history; identification of major trends; and some discussion of current issues.

U.S. Department of Health, Education and Welfare, Social Security Administration:

Estimating Your Social Security Retirement Check. HEW Publication No. (SSA) 78–10047.

How SSI Can Help. HEW Publication No. (SSA) 77–11051.

SSI for the Aged, Blind and Disabled. HEW Publication No. (SSA) 78–11000.

A Brief Explanation of Medicare. HEW Publication No. (SSA) 78–10043.

Informational pamphlets available to the public through the Social Security Administration offices, and often other public offices. A good source of reliable information on the various services offered through the Social Security Administration, in income replacement, and payment of costs of health care.

Woodruff DS, Birren JE: *Aging, Scientific Perspectives and Social Issues.* New York, D. Van Nostrand Company, 1975.

A collection of papers by contributors, dealing with aging from a variety of scientific viewpoints, as well as identifying environmental and social issues. The content provides a basic approach to understanding the various changes taking place in the person.

chapter six
social resources
of the aged

A friend is one to whom
  one may pour out
  all the contents of one's heart,
chaff and grain together,
knowing that the gentlest of hands
  will take and sift it,
keeping what is worth keeping
  and with the breath of kindness
  blow the rest away.

Arabian Proverb

OUTLINE

Human beings are social animals. In spite of unique genetic and physical characteristics, who a person is psychologically and culturally depends largely on who he or she is within his or her social milieu. The *social environment* can be defined broadly as the society at large, that is, American society, or specifically as the dialogue between two human beings. Social resources are those affective and instrumental interpersonal processes that promote a person's well-being.

This chapter will look briefly, from an historical perspective, at the larger social milieu within which the older person has lived. Then the interaction of people within their personal social systems will be examined. The relationship between people's social resources and how they cope with the stresses, challenges, and losses within the social milieu will be discussed. Social networks are important both as resources for health maintenance and as indicators of social health status.

AN HISTORICAL VIEW OF SOCIETAL FACTORS

For a nurse who is working with older clients to have some understanding of the societal influences that the older people have experienced she or he must consider the social changes that have taken place during the clients' lifetimes. Elderly people, today, have lived through more societal change in their lifetimes than several generations of their ancestors did. For example, someone who is 70 years old in 1980 was born just before the beginning of World War I. He or she was a child when the transition from buggy to car was a big event in family life. This was the time when the best way to travel was by train, there were no interstate highways, airplanes were a fairly new idea, and space travel was purely fictional. Radios were available in only a few homes, and television was still in the experimental stage. Many homes did not have electricity, and the first talking picture was not produced until 1927. Governmental support for retirement was unheard of, America was primarily rural, and the extended family usually lived in close proximity to the nuclear family.

A look at the history of the 1920s and the 1930s, which is when this client was a child and young adult, can give some impression of the vast number of social, economic, and cultural changes that have taken place during the client's lifetime.

Although the changes in the larger society have been much the same for today's older population, each person functioned in his or her own unique social network of primary and secondary relationships. The extent to which people were influenced by the occurrences and norms of the larger society was greatly influenced by the norms and experiences within their more immediate social groups. Some people who are now in the second half of life were very active in the political, educational, or social life of the local community or the wider society and, therefore, were very much a part of the changes that occurred in the larger society. Other people have lived in environments that were less affected by the broader societal changes and, as a result, have little awareness of these changes. These people, generally, have been active in a social milieu that focused on the needs and activities of the immediate group. Such people come to old age with different perceptions of societal changes and of the importance of those changes to their own lives.

Therefore, consideration of the cultural perspective and the ethnicity that is associated with these differences is important. Moreover, people who have absorbed information from their changing world, who have adapted to societal fluctuations, and who have adjusted to the changing pace of life around them are usually quite skilled in coping with life in general.

SOCIAL NETWORK THEORY

Kurt Lewin's field theory of group dynamics is important to the understanding of social and group differences (1). Lewin's theory shows that the group to which individuals belong is the primary source of their perceptions, feelings, and actions. The field theory demonstrates that there are environmental forces that impinge on or influence the person in many ways. Likewise, each person influences other people in the environment. A mechanism of interdependence and continuous movement exists between the person and the environment. Lewin's theory has provided a background for both sociological and psychological understanding of the human being.

Although the field theory seems quite comprehensive, and even holistic, it is seen by some as an impersonal theory, devoid of an adequate indication of the significance of the human component in the interaction that takes place between the person and the environment. Therefore, the social network theory has been advanced by several social scientists.

The social network theory extends Lewin's theory to focus on the personal nature of human interaction. Adams defines a person's network as "those persons with whom he maintains contact and has some form of social bonds" (2). A slightly different definition is given by Speck and Rueven, who maintain that a social network is "that group of persons who maintain an ongoing significance in each other's lives by fulfilling specific human needs" (3).

Social networks develop in human interaction because of affection, consensus, or obligation. Affection involves having an attraction for another person, a feeling of liking, or positive sentiment. Consensus refers to the sharing of common values, beliefs, goals, interests, and attitudes. Obligation refers to a reciprocity-responsibility norm, a social necessity, or a symbiotic relationship. Adams expanded the idea of obligation to a concept of "positive concern." He states "we would affirm that obligation and need, when coupled with long-term involvement and continuing interest, evolves into a positive or affectional force, which we shall label 'positive concern' " (2).

Both structural and intensity components comprise a social network. Structural elements are kin and nonkin. Other labels for the nonkin aspect of this network would be friends, neighbors, coworkers, and associates. Pattison groups these nonkin labels into a category he calls "affective kin" (4). Most sociologists divide the kin category into nuclear and extended, or primary and secondary groups, whereas the nonkin category is often perceived more generally.

The intensity categories of a social network are: *1)* intimate, *2)* effective, and *3)* nominal and are usually used in referring to the structural category of kin. However, these intensity categories should be extended to include nonkin relationships since we live in an urbanized, mobile society in which the opportunity for face-to-face encounter with kin is often minimal. For this and other reasons, many people have learned to establish intimate, meaningful relationships with nonkin of various types. Moreover, many work situations require both effective and nominal types of interactions. This is also true in relationships with neighbors and acquaintances in social and community groups. Extension of intensity categories to interactions with nonkin is supported by Adams' theory and research (2).

The intimate intensity category is characterized by frequent contact, strong attachment, and open communication. Therefore, intensity categories should apply to nonkin as well as kin in the social network, for maintaining a close relationship with another person is central to existence throughout life (5). Thus, in a situation where the traditional kinship system does not provide for intimate relationships, a person often develops intimate nonkin relationships. This process can be an especially important resource for the older person who experiences loss of close loved ones.

The effective intensity category is described as shallow attachment and shallow communication. The term *effective* itself refers to the idea of necessary service or action that may be involved in a relationship. Relationships that develop in the work setting and in social and political settings would most likely be effective in intensity.

Nominal intensity refers to the part of the social network that is mainly beyond the experience of the person in that there is minimal or nonexistent contact or involvement. This can happen in kin networks, especially in large, extended families that are far apart geographically and in life-style and interests. In the wider society, where persons are known by their position with little personal involvement, the nominal intensity category is operating (2).

Usually the primary structural category includes both intimate and effective kinds of intensity, whereas the secondary groups are likely to demonstrate effective or nominal intensity categories. In other words, a person's social network is a very important social resource throughout life and especially in old age when losses are more likely to occur. Human relationships provide support in many ways.

Nonetheless, the same relationships that are social resources are also those relationships that can result in the experience of loss. The loss of spouse, siblings, and other significant close friends and relatives is a common experience as one gets older. However, a person who has a fairly stable, and adequately sized social network has a useful resource for dealing with the losses he or she experiences. The loss of people in the primary group is usually a much more intense kind of loss than the loss of people in secondary groups. Losses in secondary groups are also significant in that they often remind people of their increasing age and make them more acutely aware of their eventual death.

The older client has developed a life-style that includes his or her established social network of interaction. The community in which a person lives is important to this network. The client who has lived in the same community all of his or her life is apt to have quite a different social network than the client who is living in a new community, whether that new community is a retirement community in the sunbelt or a new high-rise apartment building in the home town. The person who has lived in the same community throughout life is less likely to have felt the need to develop new friendships, whereas the person who has moved is much more aware of the need for new friends.

Moreover, the person whose primary social contacts have been with persons in the work environment will find a need to make new contacts and friends when employment ceases.

PURPOSE OF A SOCIAL NETWORK

People need social networks to provide both affective and instrumental support. Affective support refers to the emotional, personal, intimate kind of support that one person provides for another human being—the acceptance of the person as he or she is. Affective support is partly described by the Arabian proverb at the beginning of this chapter. People need this kind of support to meet their belonging needs (Maslow), to develop self-esteem, and to stimulate growth toward self-actualization. Affective support comes more from ascription, or who we are as persons, than from what we have achieved in life. Even though the American culture values achievement more than ascription, the affective domain of the social network is very important and is now being used as a model for psychotherapy (4, 6).

Instrumental support includes financial support, assistance with tasks, aid during emergencies, and the things that are part of "neighboring," that is, the sharing of goods and services within a community. An example of neighboring in rural America in the past was thrashing time every summer and is symbolized in today's urban setting by the classic "cup of sugar" borrowed from a neighbor.

Pattison describes a healthy social network, which he uses as a basis for the development of the Pattison Psychosocial Kinship Inventory, as having five major components.

> First, the relationship has a relatively high degree of *interaction,* whether face-to-face, by telephone, or by letter. In other words, a person invests in those with whom he has contact. Second, the relationship has a strong *emotional intensity.* The degree of investment in others is reflected in the intensity of feeling toward the other. Third, the emotion is generally *positive.* Negative relationships are maintained only when other variables force the maintenance of the relationship, such as a boss or spouse. Fourth, the relationship has an *instrumental base.* That is, not only is the other person held in positive emotional regard, but can be counted upon to provide concrete assistance. Fifth, the relationship is *symmetrically reciprocal.* That is, the other person returns the strong positive feeling, and may count upon you for instrumental assistance. There is an affective and instrumental quid pro quo (7, p.17).

NETWORK SIZE AS AN INDICATOR OF SOCIAL HEALTH

Although the findings of several other researchers and therapists are quite similar, Pattison's data will be used here as a basis for the description of the size of the social network of healthy persons. Pattison and his associates found that

> . . . the healthy person has 20 to 30 persons in his intimate psychosocial network. The relationships are rated positive on all five variables of interpersonal relations. There are typically 5 or 6 people in each sub-group of family, relatives, friends, neighbors, and work or social contacts. About half to two-thirds of these people have social relations with each other, so that the social connectedness ratio is about 60%. Friends are the most highly valued members of the network outside of the nuclear family, and are most often sought for effective and instrumental assistance. Significant relations are found in multiple areas of life interaction, and the social matrix is semi-open to other people. In summary, the normal person has a finite primary group of about 25 people, who comprise a stable yet not exclusive psychosocial system (7, pp. 18–19).

Pattison goes on to say they found that the neurotic population in their study had only 10 to 12 people in their social network, and the psychotic population in the study had only four or five people in their psychosocial network.

SETTINGS IN WHICH NETWORKS ARE ESTABLISHED

Bossevain gives examples in other cultures of rather large social networks and shows that the longer a person lives, the higher the number of people in his network is likely to be (8). With the mobility and increasing complexity of American culture, it is not uncommon for people to develop intimate relationships with other people in various places where they have lived. When people move from a community in which they have a good social network in operation, it is not expected that a high degree of interaction or instrumental and reciprocal relationships will continue with the majority of the people who are left behind. However, it is not uncommon for a person or family to maintain an intimate, positive, and meaningful relationship with one or several of the people who live in the old community. The degree of interaction is maintained by telephone, letter, and by occasional visits. The reasons for the continuation of the interaction are most likely related to the strength of the emotional intensity that existed in the relationship before the geographic change. In looking at the intensity category, which was described earlier, the relationship that is likely to continue after geographic relocation takes place is the relationship that is described as intimate, especially in respect to the affection and consensus aspects of the relationship.

What then are the common settings within a community in which intimate social networks are established? Beyond the intimate relationships that are established with kin, both nuclear and extended, the settings in which relationships are established vary somewhat with the type of community that is involved. Social institutions such as place of employment, the educational system, and the community structure have already been mentioned. In addition, the religious system, that is, church or synagogue, in which a person and his family are involved is often an important locale for establishment of an intimate social network. The degree of one's involvement in religion will, of course, determine the significance of this social institution in the development of social networks.

The settings where social contacts take place can be seen as social resources for the older person. When a person retires the work setting is often no longer available as a resource for establishing social contacts. A person may maintain friendships that were established at work, but the establishment of new friendships within that setting is unlikely. Beyond the resources that the family makes available, communities have varying degrees of established activities and organizations that provide a resource for the development of social networks for the older person. Senior citizens centers, Golden Age Clubs, congregate meal sites, recreation centers, and service clubs are some of the resources available in many communities.

A National Council on Aging, Louis Harris Associates Public Opinion Study, which was published in 1976, reveals some interesting information about the kinds of activities in which people who are over 65 are engaged compared with what the total public thinks most people over 65 spend their time doing. Of the total public polled, 67% said that people over 65 spend much time watching television, whereas in the over-65 population only 36% said that they spent a lot of time watching television. On the other hand, in the category of "participating in fraternal or community organizations or clubs" only 17% of the people over 65 said they spent a lot of time in this activity, whereas 26% of the total public thought that the people over 65 spent much time in club activities. The item that was ranked the highest by the people over 65 was "socializing with friends." Only 31% of the people over 65 said they spent a lot of time "sitting and thinking" but 62% of the total public thought that is how people over 65 spend most of their time.

It is interesting to note in this survey that people over 65, were not greatly involved in the activities available to them. For instance, ranking very low were "participating in fraternal or community organizations and clubs," "working part time or full time," "doing volunteer work," "participating in political activities," and "participating in sports such as golfing, swimming and tennis." Ranking higher for the person over 65 were activities that were not likely to be social in nature such as gardening or raising plants, reading, watching television, and sitting and thinking (9).

This information is not conclusive and, again, points not only to the heterogeneity of the older population but also to the importance of ascertaining clients' perceptions of the adequacy of their social involvement when assessment is being done.

Social resources are important to people who are confronted with the natural changes that are the result of the contraction of the family and social mobility, which often moves children and grandchildren away from grandparents. Social resources are also needed to help people deal with the losses that come with the illness and death of others who are important to them.

Social resources should not be seen as ends in themselves. Holistic assessment requires that the nurse consider the social resources in balance with the psychological resources that the person is using. It may be that a person does not chose to replace a loss by developing a new social contact. If the client seems exceptionally withdrawn from interaction with others, it may be necessary to assess whether he or she is still in an early stage of the grieving process (10). Providing opportunities for clients to verbalize feelings about losses they have experienced may not only facilitate the assessment process for the nurse but may also give clients an opportunity to examine their feelings about the losses and help them to find their own resolution of the losses. It is possible for a person to be coping effectively with a loss while still remembering and frequently thinking about the person who has died, especially if the relationship was a long, meaningful one.

However, ascertaining the client's wishes and making him or her aware of resources that are available is an important role of the nurse.

In summary, social resources available to the older person are the people in the person's social network, the activities in which he or she is involved, alone or with others, and the religious milieu in which the client functions, which includes both significant people and other resources. In addition, the community structures that have been established in response to the Conferences on Aging and federal and state laws are social resources that are available to the older person.

MALE/FEMALE DIFFERENCES IN USE
OF THE SOCIAL NETWORK

There is evidence that women tend to develop more intimate relationships in their social networks than men do. Whether or not this is related to the sociological observation that men are more instrumental, that is, more involved in doing, and women are more affective, or more concerned with being, is not clear. The behavioral norms that are culture specific may also be important here. In the American culture, children are taught from infancy that boys are strong, unemotional, and productive; whereas girls may cry and be more concerned with the emotional components of life. It is possible that an explanation of the phenomenon of women having more intimate interaction than men relates to the fact that in the middle years, and as the second half of life begins, men more often than women are very busy and involved in their work or professional life and have less time for the establishment of intimate relationships outside the kinship system. It may be that the men's priorities are financial security rather than affective security. Although many women are in the work force, more women seem to take the time to establish intimate relationships within the neighborhood or elsewhere. The fact that women are primarily responsible in American culture for the rearing of the children may be an important point here, too. For example, neighbor women are likely to babysit for each other for short periods of time and thus establish both an intimate and effective relationship. This kind of responsibility and interaction is less likely to be assumed by the men in the community.

Whatever the reason, research has shown that more women than men have *confidants*, that is, people with whom they have intimate relationships (5). This fact, along with the fact that a woman's role does not change as much as a man's role at retirement, may speak to the greater difficulty men have in finding fulfillment in retirement. This may also provide support for the idea that women can cope with widowhood more effectively than men can. Solving the broader societal problem of male/female differences that relate to their social network systems cannot be done when a person reaches the second half of life. However, it would seem that health professionals have some responsibility to provide opportunities and information to both men and women about available social resources. A better solution probably would be for men and women to establish at an earlier age a broad base of activity and interaction so when they reach retirement they will have both personal and social resources that can improve their ability to cope with personal and social losses.

USE OF THE SOCIAL NETWORK

A person's social network can be used both to foster and to facilitate independence during the second half of life. An assessment of a client's current social network is useful so when he or she must face a challenge or stress in which he or she needs assistance, the resource of the social network can be brought into play. Persons who are healthy can rather quickly become ill, either physically or mentally, and either chronically or critically. In any of these situations, a certain amount of dependency occurs because of the limitations imposed by the illness. Knowledge of the client's network at such a time provides an important resource to help the client to return to a healthy state or to optimum functioning with continued limitations.

Assessment of a network can be done in a one-to-one interaction with the client, or it can be done with the client's network in a network session (11). In the one-to-one situation, the client can state or list the people who are currently in his or her primary network structure and who provide affective and instrumental support. These persons may be kin or nonkin, or both. The client can also list people who, although not currently active in the client's primary group, could potentially be important resources within the network, especially when specific problems arise.

There are times when initiating a network session with a client's primary network group is necessary; however, if a client is healthy, the need for such a meeting would be unlikely. Such a meeting would be more essential at a time when specific problems need to be discussed and solved. At those times, the nurse can assist the client in convening a meeting of his or her network group. If the problem is a mental health one, the nurse would most likely work with a psychiatric social worker, a psychiatrist, and/or a psychologist in setting up such a meeting. Extreme loneliness would be an example of such a problem. On the other hand, if the problem is primarily physical in nature—such as, being too weak to cook, to shop, and to take care of the house, the nurse would more likely work with a social worker, homemaker, and/or the physician along with people in the primary group.

It should be pointed out here that the social network as a resource is not a substitute for community services and organizations. It is just one more approach to meeting needs that exist among the elderly in any community. Collaboration with other people and organizations is an important component of effective use of available resources, as well as of meeting the needs of the clients in the best possible way. An attitude of competition among community groups working with and for the elderly does not promote effective coordination of available services for the clients.

When an assessment of a client's social network is done, either with the client or in a network session, several items need to be identified. First, how self-sufficient is the client—physically, psychologically, socially, and economically? Second, what is the network's ability to provide the affective and/or instrumental support that the client needs or may need in the near future? Third, what are the stresses or challenges that the client is facing and that the network is dealing with at this time? Fourth, what client, network, and professional resources can be best used to meet the challenge(s) the client is now facing (11)?

AGED PERSONS AS SOCIAL RESOURCES

In Chapter 1, it was stated that "aging has become more of a social problem than a social resource," and that the aged "have been leaders in family and community life for many years." These statements, along with the premise that chronological age is not an indicator of deteriorating abilities and with the substantial support in literature and experience for seeing older persons as having a broad range of experience and knowledge that can be useful to others in the society, leads to the assertion that the aged *are* a social resource. Their experience gained from living, their experience and knowledge gained from their professional and/or work life, their special knowledge about many kinds of tasks and activities, and their "long view of time" perspective, makes the elderly in a community resources for themselves, their peers, and for the next generation(s).

Erikson's suggestion that a child learns trust by interacting with an adult who displays ego integrity points to the important contribution that grandparents and their peers can make in relating to grandchildren. The notion that it is the role of grandparents to "spoil" grandchildren may be based on the frustration that parents experience because they may not yet have achieved a calmness and equanimity about their own goals and roles in life that comes with ego integrity. Disparaging comments about grandparent/grandchild relationships may come from feelings of loss that parents can have about missing some of the joy and sharing that they observe taking place in the grandparent/grandchild relationship. Often grandparents are more acceptant of creative exploration in grandchildren than are parents, thus freeing children to develop and to grow emotionally, socially, and intellectually. Even in the American culture, grandchildren can learn something about their roots and sources of identity with history and the future through interactions with grandparents.

Being a grandparent is probably the most "socially acceptable" way that an older person can use the resource of "self" in relation to others. The importance of these relationships should not be minimized, however, this is not the only sharing of "self" that is important for the older person.

A fair number of older people, for a variety of reasons, do not have consanguineous grandchildren. How can they then function in the role of grandparent? There are many opportunities for these people to have grandparent-type relationships with members of the coming generation(s). They can serve as volunteers in foster grandparent programs, work in nursery schools, tutor children with special needs, and work in other settings where interaction between the young and the old can be mutually beneficial.

Moreover, grandparenting is not the only meaningful way for older persons to share themselves with others. Furthermore, some people who are in the second half of life may not view "grandparenting" as a role they would select. In such situations, it is important for the nurse not to assume that there is a problem. What is the client's perspective? What are his or her priorities in life? Does he or she believe that life is full and meaningful without the "socially acceptable" grandparent role? It is quite possible, that when the whole person is considered, certain notions about what people "must" or "ought" to do or want will need to be laid aside.

Although others may see older persons as resources, the people themselves may choose not to function in social settings or to share themselves. Again, the person has a right to make such a choice. Holistic assessment should aid in determining if the person truly wishes to remain somewhat isolated or if he or she takes this stance because of previous disappointing and painful relationships with other persons.

There are times when older people would like to share themselves with others in the community, but they are not aware of the opportunities for such sharing. It would be appropriate to provide information to clients, after assessment, about organized and other ways for older people to be involved in social and community settings. Loneliness is often a social problem for older people, especially in a society where roles are compartmentalized and the pace of life is accelerated. Often a holistic approach to assessment can discover loneliness before it has caused severe depression or withdrawal, and intervention, using the actual and potential social network, can occur.

Sometimes the process of reminiscence and life review stimulates persons to start writing about their thoughts, feelings, experiences, and observations. The knowledge and wisdom that they share through the written word can provide personal fulfillment and be another approach to intergenerational communication.

SUMMARY

Even when it appears, based on information about healthy people and their social networks, that an older person has a need in the social resources category; this information must be considered in conjunction with cultural, physical, psychological, and economic data about the client. When seen in its totality, what first appeared to be a social need may actually be a coping strategy that the client has developed and does not wish to change at this time. This possibility should not, however, influence nurses to be superficial in assessment or to be quick to make inferences before adequate data have been collected.

Data collection with older clients is often quite time consuming because they usually have longer histories and have had many experiences that may be significant data to the holistic assessment. Nevertheless, extreme verbosity during history taking and physical examination may be a demonstration that clients have unmet social needs, and that they are using this opportunity to meet needs for social contact. The nurse should be sensitive to this possibility but should also clearly state the purpose of the health assessment process to the client so unrealistic expectations are not developed. If a client seems to be using the assessment time as a way to meet social needs, the nurse should seek more specific data about how the client is meeting social needs and tell the client that she or he will help the client to find other resources when the initial assessment phase of the interaction is concluded.

REFERENCES

1. Lewin K: *Field Theory in Social Science.* New York, Harper & Bros, 1951.
2. Adams BN: Interaction theory and the social network. *Sociometry:* 30:64–78, 1967.
3. Speck RV, Rueveni U: Network therapy—a developing concept. *Family Process* 8:182–191, 1969.
4. Pattison EM: Social system psychotherapy. *American J Psychother* 27:396–409, 1973.
5. Lowenthal MF, Haven C: Interaction and adaptation: intimacy as a critical variable, in Neugarten, BL: *Middle Age and Aging.* Chicago, The University of Chicago Press, 1968, pp. 390–400.
6. Speck RV, Attneave CL: *Family Networks.* New York, Pantheon Books, 1973.
7. Pattison EM: A Theoretical-Empirical Base for Social Systems Therapy. Symposium presented at the 33rd Annual Conference of the American Group Psychotherapy Association, February 1976, Boston, Massachusetts.
8. Boissevain J: *Friends of Friends: Networks, Manipulators and Coalitions.* New York, St. Martin's Press, 1974.
9. Setlow C: *Aging in America: Implications for Society.* Washington, DC, The National Council on the Aging, 1976.
10. Kubler-Ross E: *On Death and Dying.* New York, Macmillan Company, 1969.
11. Garrison JE, Howe J: Community intervention with the elderly: a social network approach, *J Am Geriatr Soc* 24:329–333, 1976.

ANNOTATED BIBLIOGRAPHY

Boissevain J: *Friends of Friends.* New York, St. Martin's Press, 1974.
    A cross-cultural view of networks using the author's structural diagrams and formulas in evaluation.
Kubler-Ross E: *On Death and Dying.* New York, Macmillan Company, 1969.
    Excellent concise resource on the grief stages involved with dying and death. Useful to anyone who works with persons who are terminally ill.

Mennell SJ: *Sociological Theory: Uses and Unities.* New York, Praeger Publishers, 1974.

An overview of sociological theory and its relationship to social research. States views of various social scientists clearly and concisely.

Phillips DC: *Holistic Thought in Social Science.* Stanford, Calif, Stanford University Press, 1976.

A philosophical and theoretical basis for a holistic approach to people and their systems is presented.

Speck RV, Attneave CL: *Family Networks.* New York, Pantheon Books, 1973.

The authors share from their own personal experience in social networks and discuss the therapeutic use of network intervention, especially in the field of mental health.

chapter seven
holistic nursing assessment of the healthy aged

The purpose of clinical nursing is "to facilitate the efforts of the individual to overcome the obstacles which currently interfere with his ability to respond capably to demands made of him by his condition, environment, situation and time."

Ernestine Wiedenbach
Clinical Nursing: A Helping Art
New York: Springer Publishing
Company, Inc., 1964

OUTLINE

Since several excellent books focus on the total nursing process and explain it in detail, an extensive discussion is not included here. Rather, specific emphasis is placed on phase one of the nursing process, that is, on *holistic assessment* (1–3). In this chapter, some general statements about assessment will be made, and some examples of application of an assessment tool will be given.

Even though there are many useful outlines and approaches to either compartmentalized or holistic assessment, a tool that the nurse develops for him or herself is usually much more useful to the individual nurse. Use of one's own scientific knowledge base and philosophy about the nature of humans and the purpose of nursing provides the background for individualized development of assessment tools. Moreover, the personal analysis and synthesis that occurs in the development of a holistic assessment tool tends to internalize the components of the assessment process more effectively than does the use of a tool that someone else has developed.

Up to this point in this book, examples and practical applications that have been given have been fragmented instances that have usually related only to one area of the client's situation or characteristics. In this chapter, a pragmatic methodology for assessing the whole person efficiently and accurately is presented.

In 1973 the American Nurses' Association published *Standards of Nursing Practice,* a useful guide to application of the nursing process (4). Standard I states "The collection of data about the health status of the client/patient is systematic and continuous. The data are accessible, communicated, and recorded." The outcome of this systematic data collection is stated in Standard II, "Nursing diagnoses are derived from health status data." These brief statements provide a basis for discussing nursing assessment.

Any comprehensive health/nursing assessment attempts to place the client at some point on the health/illness continuum. To do this in a holistic manner, the client's present environment and culture and his or her past and present experiences are important. The nurse can best proceed through the assessment process by an integrated use of generalized naturalistic observations, health history data, and a physical examination of the client.

NURSE-CLIENT INTERACTION DURING ASSESSMENT

When the nurse first meets the client, an adequate introduction is essential to the establishment of an interaction that promotes the client's participation in assessment.

Therapeutic communication skills need to be developed by the nurse so the primary focus of the assessment interaction is the client and his or her needs. Knowing that a helping relationship comprises several phases provides the basis for a nurse to develop communication techniques that are sensitive to the client's verbal and nonverbal information. Therapeutic communication is also an important technique in the nursing intervention component of the nursing process.

The preinteraction phase of a helping relationship is the time when the nurse prepares for a first interaction with a client. During the introductory phase, the nurse and client identify themselves to each other and establish the purpose and proposed duration of the relationship. The length of the working phase of the interaction varies, depending on the goals that have been established and on the current needs of the client. Successful termination of a relationship is important and should include a summary of accomplishments and closure of the relationship. Effective use of the phases of a helping relationship is important to each new nurse-client relationship (1).

The nurse comes to the assessment interaction with respect for the client's rights to physical and psychological privacy and for other contingencies that may be infringing on the client's time and needs. The nurse should observe for both verbal and nonverbal cues from the client, which will indicate the client's degree of comfort in the situation and willingness to proceed with the assessment. The most effective sequencing of the components of the assessment process involves meeting the client and collecting some information, usually called history taking, from the client before the physical examination component of the assessment.

Although the length of time that a history and physical examination should take depends in part on the amount of time available, sufficient time should be allotted so adequate consideration can be given to the whole person as he or she interacts with the current environment.

COLLECTION OF SUBJECTIVE DATA

The sample questions that follow are not all inclusive; however, they are intended to show the kinds of questions that can be used to collect information about the various aspects of a person's health status.

What are the general kinds of information that need to be collected during a nursing assessment? First, what are the cultural variables involved? Do the clients' beliefs about health and their status as older people parallel the beliefs of the nurse? Or, are there significant differences that the nurse should ascertain so he or she can understand the clients' related behaviors and practices more completely? Are there ethnic traditions or beliefs that vary remarkably from the expectations that the health care system might place on clients? Are there beliefs about disease causation, folk methods of cure, or dietary habits that disagree with what may be prescribed by the health care professionals? Such information is essential to a clear perception of each client's health status.

Second, how do clients describe their physical status? Do they see themselves as healthy? How do they view the nonpathological physical changes of aging? Has the reality of physical aging resulted in changes in rest, activity, or nutritional behavior? If so, do the clients see these changes as normal and incidental? Or have the changes been disruptive forces in their lives?

The nurse's general naturalistic observations, starting from the moment the interaction begins, often provide the basis for further questions. Observations that the nurse makes about gait, posture, and movement of each client can provide important cues for specific questions about physical health. The information collected during history taking provides important data for specific components of the physical assessment. The clients' physical examinations are an important part of assessing their physical health and can be carried out more effectively if the nurse is aware of the clients' perceptions of their state of health and their reports of challenges or problems they face.

Assessing the psychological health of an older person does not lend itself to the discovery of as much objective data as does the evaluation of physical health. However, a person's attitude about self, personal health, and abilities has a remarkable influence on how challenges are met and on what coping strategies are developed. The locus of control construct might be a useful tool to discover a client's perception about who is in charge of his or her life. That is, does the client have primarily an internal or an external locus of control? This kind of information can be useful in discovering the client's expectations of the role of health care professionals. For instance, the client who is externally controlled may attribute the responsibility for his or her health or illness to others rather than to any personal behaviors and may be less likely to follow interventions as instructed. Both Peck's and Erikson's descriptions of the psychological health of the mature adult can be useful guidelines to the nurse in evaluating the psychological health of a client. An example of one way to use these tools is covered in the sample assessment outlined in this chapter. Is the client basically satisfied with who he or she is as a thinking, feeling, sexual being? Or, does the client express regret or feelings of incompleteness because of not having certain psychological needs fulfilled?

Do the client's economic resources adequately meet his or her daily needs? Does he or she feel economic resources are adequate or is he or she experiencing poverty? Is the client aware of and using all the economic resources available through the current federal and state laws?

Does the client eagerly share information about social interaction with the people who are significant to him or her, or is the client hesitant to speak about kin and friends? Does he or she refer to persons in his or her social networks? Does the client speak of relationships with these persons as being primarily rewarding and meaningful, or is there a reluctance to comment on people in his or her social networks? Do the people in the client's social networks meet affectional and instrumental needs? Who are these people?

Does the client express a sense of self-worth and of belonging? Are examples given of things that make life meaningful and enjoyable or is the primary focus of the conversation on losses and the inadequacy of the present life situation?

The preceding questions may seem like a random selection, but they are the kinds of things the nurse needs to think through when a holistic approach to assessment is undertaken. The apparent randomness of these questions points to the need for a useful tool to bring coherent structure to the assessment. Structure is needed not only to streamline the process but also to ensure the inclusion of all the important components of assessment. There is no one absolutely correct or best tool. There are many tools, published and unpublished, used by nurses and other professionals that can be incorporated or adapted into the repertoire of the nurse who is developing his or her own assessment approaches.

AN EXAMPLE OF A MULTIDIMENSIONAL ASSESSMENT TOOL

In the mid-70s, Eric Pfeiffer and his associates at the Duke University Center for the Study of Aging and Human Development developed a comprehensive assessment tool, which can be viewed as an excellent guide for collection of subjective data from a client. Since the goals of their project included assessment of resources and services to older persons, the questionnaire goes beyond what is required for individual assessment. It is, however, easily adapted to use with individual clients and has been used effectively in this way.

The questionnaire is well organized, easy to follow, and includes the categories covering the following areas: social resources, economic resources, mental health, physical health, and activities of daily living (5). A numerical rating scale has been designed for each category as well as a cumulative score. This tool can be used as a guide for collection of nursing history data; however, it needs to be supplemented by physical examination if client assessment is to be complete.

DEVELOPING A TOOL: AN EXAMPLE

Developing a generalized holistic nursing assessment tool is not an easy task since individualization is important for both the nurse and the client. Logical sequencing of categories and questions for one nurse may seem awkward and disorganized for another nurse. Also, the client may come to the interaction with a need or concern that he or she needs to discuss before a detailed, holistic assessment can occur. Sensitivity to such needs is important, and the assessment process should be adapted accordingly. This adaptation can occur without losing a holistic approach with the client. The sequence of categories in the sample outline below is not as important as the effort to be holistic and concise. The length of the sample may indicate that conciseness was not considered; however, the goal to be both complete and concise in assessment outlines remains a challenge to nursing and other health professions.

A Sample Nursing Assessment Data Collection Outline

This outline includes cultural, physical, psychological, social and economic assessment. The data are primarily subjective, that is, they are told by the client to the nurse in an interview.

Outline	*Category and Explanation*
A. *Demographic data*	Necessary general information
Name, age, sex, marital status.	
address, telephone number, occu-	Social
pation, name(s) of primary health	
care provider(s)	

Outline   *Category and Explanation*

B. *Health-illness data*

1. Belief: define health; define   Cultural
   illness
2. Own physical health status: Physical—such as: chills, sweats,
   description of current, recent   weakness, fatigue, weight change
   changes in
3. Compare own health status   Cultural, social and psychological
   with that of others in age
   group
4. Health practices: rest, activity, Physical; also is often cultural, psy-
   nutrition, drugs, immuniza-   chological or social
   tions, habits
5. Specific health problems
   (past and present)

   · Allergies—food and drugs   Physical
   · Integumentary
   · Sensory—touch, vision,
     hearing, smelling, tasting
   · Gastrointestinal—dental
     health, ingestion, digestion,
     and elimination
   · Cardiopulmonary—diseases,
     symptoms (shortness of
     breath, pain, cough), activity
     change (ordered by physician
     or self-imposed)
   · Breasts—changes, practice
     of self-examination
   · Musculoskeletal—pain,
     weakness, swelling, cramps,
     fractures, stiffness
   · Neurological—tremors, diz-
     ziness, depression
   · Genitourinary—pain, fre-
     quency, difficulty starting
     stream, bleeding, inconti-
     nence

C. *Psychological health data*   According to Peck
                                         Psychological
   1. Ego differentiation   (For the purpose of clarity specific
                                         questions are used as examples
      · Do you enjoy life now?   here.)

Outline   *Category and Explanation*

    · What kinds of things bring
      joy?

    · Does life seem to get better   First three questions similar to
      or worse for you?   Neugarten et al—zest category

    · How did you adjust to re-
      tirement?

    · What creative activities do   Similar to Maslow's metaneeds
      you participate in?

  2. Body transcendence

    · How do you feel when you   Neugarten et al—mood tone category
      notice that your body is get-
      ting older?

    · What do you do to cope with   Neugarten et al—mood tone and
      the aging process?   fortitude/resolution

    · Does physical activity influ-   Neugarten et al—Self-concept
      ence your self concept? How?

  3. Ego transcendence

    · How satisfied are you with   Neugarten et al—mood tone
      your accomplishments in
      life?

    · How is your belief system a   Cultural (religious)
      resource to you?

    · Have most of your goals been   Similar to internal locus of control
      achieved in the past?

    · What are some of your goals   Neugarten et al—goal congruence
      for the future?   and fortitude/resolution

    · What do you see as your role   Neugarten et al—self-concept
      in relation to younger
      people?

    · How have you dealt with   Neugarten et al—fortitude/resolution
      death of people you care
      about?

  4. In general terms, how would
    you describe your personality?

D. *Economic resource data*

  1. Income   Economic and social

Outline   *Category and Explanation*

    · Change in past five years
    · Adequacy to meet basic
      needs—food, shelter, cloth-
      ing
    · Adequacy for desired
      goals—"splurge", trips, re-
      creation, entertaining, do-
      nations

2. Resources shared by others   Social, cultural
   with client
3. Housing   Economic

    · Quality—space, heat, secu-
      rity, etc.
    · Privacy
    · Client satisfaction with
      housing
    · Proximity to activites of
      choice   Social

4. Neighborhood   Social

    · Client satisfaction   Psychological
    · Security
    · Is it a good place   Cultural
      for older people?

E. *Cultural and social data*

1. Client perception of own status
   and respect within own social
   network   Cultural
2. Who is in client's social network? family, neighbors,   Social
   friends?

    · To whom would client go for
      affective or instrumental as-
      sistance?
    · Frequency of interaction
      with persons in network
      (daily, weekly, monthly—
      with number of persons)

Outline   *Category and Explanation*

   3. Reciprocity of relationships

     · For whom is client an affec-   Cultural and social
      tive or instrumental re-
      source?

     · Does client have at least one
      confidant?

   4. Participation in groups/
     organizations, organized and
     casual

     · Frequency   Social and cultural
     · Adequacy

While taking the client's history and conducting the physical examination, the nurse should use language and explanations that the client can understand. For instance, a client is not likely to know the meaning of "instrumental assistance"; therefore, descriptive, concrete methods should be used to explain the concept. Examples of questions about this topic are "If you needed help with some housekeeping activities, who would you ask to help you?" or "If you needed transportation to the grocery store, on whom would you call?"

THE PHYSICAL EXAMINATION

The outline given below is abbreviated and does not provide any guidance about technique. More detailed outlines and specific instructions about examination techniques can be found elsewhere (6,7). The physical examination provides data that are primarily objective. An integrated, systematic head-to-toe examination is usually the most efficient approach to physical examination. The client needs of physical privacy, warmth, and comfort should be met throughout the examination.

Outline for Physical Examination

   1. *General observations:* posture, gait, body movement, personal hygiene, speech patterns

2. *Weight, height, vital signs*
3. *Vision (bilaterally):* condition of eyes and eyelids; color of sclera and conjunctiva; pupil size, shape, equality, and response; lens transparency; muscle function; visual acuity; visual fields
4. *Hearing (bilaterally):* gross auditory acuity, ear canal and tympanic membrane condition
5. *Nose:* symmetry, patency, olfactory ability bilaterally
6. *Mouth and oropharynx:* condition of hard and soft palate, tongue, gums, salivary glands, uvula, oropharynx; teeth—condition (fractures, caries), number of natural teeth, use of prostheses
7. *Head and neck:* symmetry of features, freedom of movement, lesions lymph node enlargement, carotid pulses
8. *Breasts and axillae:* symmetry of size, shape, color and surface characteristics, masses
9. *Respiration:* thorax—diameters, configuration, respiratory pattern, skin condition, expansion; breath sounds and vocal resonance—all lung fields
10. *Circulation:* apical/radial pulse comparison, precordial pulsations, heart sounds at all valve locations, peripheral pulses
11. *Abdomen:* contour, skin condition, movement-pulsation, peristalsis, respiration, peristaltic and vascular sounds, organ size, areas of tenderness
12. *Musculoskeletal:* torso, upper and lower extremities—contour and symmetry, muscle strength and joint function, pain, tenderness, edema
13. *Neurological:* coordination, balance, reflexes, sensory activity, function of cranial nerves

DATA ANALYSIS AND THE NURSING DIAGNOSIS

After nursing assessment data have been collected from a client, the data need to be analyzed, and the nursing diagnoses need to be made. Little and Carnevali state that the nursing diagnosis is a "concise, precise, neutral statement of client response to a stressor or potential stressor in the health area and an identification of the area(s) of impact on his lifestyle" (2). Although nurses and physicians often work closely together in meeting client needs, a nursing diagnosis is not synonymous with a medical diagnosis. Medical diagnosis focuses on disease process identification and treatment, whereas nursing diagnosis focuses on client perceptions and coping strategies in relationship to stressors. A nursing diagnosis is the last step of the assessment phase of the nursing process and the basis for client-care goals and the planning of nursing interventions. However, nursing assessment does not stop with the diagnosis, for the nursing process is ongoing. Assessment continues as long as the nurse is responsible for the care of a client.

The nursing diagnoses need to be stated concisely, although the data on which the diagnoses are based may be rather detailed. Terminology used in diagnosis statements needs to be objective and unambiguous. Little and Carnevali outline the three components of a nursing diagnosis as: *1)* "the area(s) and nature of the coping deficit(s)"; *2)* "the area of impact on day to day living and/or desired lifestyle"; and *3)* "the stressor that is the major contributor to the deficit (this may be a more optional component at times)" (2, p.156). For example, a diagnosis could be stated in an outline format.

Coping deficit

· Impairment of mobility

Impact on life-style

· Unable to take daily mile walk
· Needs to use walker in house
· Cannot go to grocery store

Major stressor

· Joint pain and stiffness in lower extremities

TWO CASE STUDIES: EXAMPLES OF HOLISTIC ASSESSMENT

The two case studies below show how a holistic history outline can be used to collect data. Neither case study should be viewed as "typical" but as an example of "healthy" older people who are facing some challenges and coping deficits for which some health care assistance is recommended. The data in the histories are presented in a modified outline style, without use of complete sentences. This demonstrates one approach to making concise brief statements while maintaining completeness and some use of client's own terminology.

Case Study

A. *Demographic data*
    J. G.; 79; male; married; lives in small rural town; retired farmer; primary health care provider is family practice physician; last visit two months ago.

B. *Health-illness data*
   Health: "feeling good"; illness: "being down on your back and being waited on." Is "pretty healthy," but "I get tired more quickly now than a month ago." Compared with peers, "I'm better off than a lot of people, because all that's wrong with me is a few achey joints."

1. Health practices: seven hours of sleep a night, half-hour to hour nap after lunch; has difficulty falling asleep the first couple nights on a trip; regular activity includes daily 10-block round-trip walk to post office, on nice days rides bicycle several miles, and gardens in the summer. He doesn't go out when it's icy and cold. Nutritional habits are controlled by wife who does most of the cooking and his 24-hour recall of intake reflects an adequate diet based on the recommended dietary allowances for his age and sex. Says his wife always has him eat his vegetables! He takes an occasional aspirin for joint pain and is on a maintainance dose of Digoxin daily. He has been on this dosage for five years at which time he was diagnosed with an irregular heart beat. He has not participated in flu vaccination programs but has had tetanus shots in the past (last one five years ago) and participated in the polio vaccination program in the 1960s. He has a glass or two of his homemade wine several times a week. He has never smoked—"Oh, a celebration cigar now and then when I'm out with the boys."

2. Specific health problems: He has no known allergies; says his skin is very dry, but he's "too lazy to use lotion regularly." Reports no sensory changes except that he thinks he's not seeing as well as he should and plans to see the ophthalmologist soon. His teeth have always been in good shape. He has no known gastrointestinal problems and states, "and I don't worry about my bowels like I'm supposed to, but I pretty much have a regular movement every other day." When he had "that problem" with his heart five years ago, he experienced "a funny feeling" in his chest but didn't really have pain. He slowed his activity on his own until he saw the doctor that time. He has maintained same activity level since then. He said he didn't realize that men should do a breast self-examination but thinks maybe it would be a good idea. He also thinks he would notice if a lump developed, because "I'm aware of my body and how it changes." He has occasional pain and stiffness, especially in knees and ankles, but believes it would be worse if he weren't active. Sometimes he gets dizzy if he moves quickly. He had severe difficulty starting his urinary stream 10 years ago, was examined, and had surgery. Has had no problems since.

C. *Psychological health data*

1. Ego differentiation: enjoys life, gets a kick out of visiting with friends, neighbors, children and grandchildren. Says it took him about a year to adjust to retirement and the extra free time but now time is filled in with "all kinds of fun things," like macrame, painting, long camping trips, refinishing furniture. Says life is better for him than it was in the past "because I just am more aware of all the things that are happening inside and around me, and it's exciting to be alive."

2. Body transcendence: says that his body getting older doesn't bother him too much now, but "it really hit me hard about 30 years ago when I suddenly realized my stamina wasn't as good as it had been. And I started getting bald then, too." But he says "I finally figured out bald men have just as much fun. It helped too when I convinced my wife that it made me more sexy." He chuckled and winked at this point. States "if I couldn't go out and walk every day and do the kinds of things I want to do, it would make me feel 'pretty down.' Like last winter, I was penned up in the house for three days, and I started not liking myself, yelling at my wife, and paced up and down thinking of all the things that are wrong with me. I'd be a grumpy invalid."

3. Ego transcendence: says he is satisfied with his accomplishments in life; says that there was a period in his life when his church didn't mean much to him but that has changed—knowing the resource of friends and a feeling of closeness to God is important to him. "This all started meaning more to me when my brother and two sisters died. I got to thinking about the future, and it makes sense inside, but I can't explain it to you now." Goals for the future include a camping trip to the northwest, a winter cruise and some time in southern California. He plans to return home in time to plant a garden. Role with younger people: his children seek his advice, as do his grandchildren; he enjoys watching his grandchildren become adults. Thinks maybe his children follow his advice too closely at times.

4. Own description of personality: "I'm a pretty neat guy, a little pig-headed sometimes, I love to kid around—drives my wife crazy, but she still likes to cuddle with me."

D. *Economic resource data*

1. Income: hasn't changed much in past five years; big change was at retirement 10 years ago, when income was cut in half. Has a

couple investments; income is adequate for basic needs and for trips if he plans carefully.
2. Shared resources: no financial support from others; gifts from family members.
3. Housing: "nice little three-bedroom, convenient, private" likes distance to post office because it "motivates" him to get exercise.
4. Neighborhood: good neighborhood, nice town, "there's only one thing wrong with this little town—everybody knows everything about everybody else—that's no good if you want privacy, but I guess it's ok if you need help." Good place for old people, about 30% of population are retired.

E. *Cultural and social data*
He is respected—"the family comes to the old man for advice—I ask them for advice too." Network: children, grandchildren, wife; neighbor next door, two couples with whom he and wife play games, visit, look at pictures, etc., about once a week; small group at church—12 people in group; visit children once a year—son, here; daughter, 100 miles away; daughter—"halfway across the country"; whole family gets together once a year usually several days at a "woodsy place, camping, and having a good time." He is a resource for wife, children, grandchildren, two couples they spend a lot of time with, and for two brothers-in-law when his sisters died, "we hurt together." Wife is confidant for most things; she consults him about things she doesn't understand. He has a "best buddy" with whom he "clears the air sometimes."

F. *Physical examination*
Mr. J.G.'s physical examination revealed mostly normal findings. There were no apparent visual problems, but he should still see eye doctor on basis of his subjective evaluation. His pulse was slightly irregular—an irregular irregularity—rate of 68. He had some joint stiffness and could not do full range of motion in his shoulders, his hips, and his ankles. He has vibratory sensory loss in toes of right foot, however, circulation is adequate.

G. *Nursing Diagnosis*
Although several potential problems exist, the subjective assessment of visual difficulty, some pulse irregularity, joint stiffness, lower extremity sensory loss, Mr. J.G. is taking steps to deal with these factors by planning to see the eye-doctor, by routine visits every three months to his family physician, and by getting regular exercise. He was advised to tell the doctor about the increased weakness he has experienced for past month. For these reasons the

nursing diagnosis for him is simply: NO PROBLEM EXISTS AT PRESENT TIME.

It is not surprising that a nurse will not find problems when doing holistic assessment with healthy aged persons. Mr. J.G. probably fits into the category of privileged aged, as outlined in Chapter 1.

Case Study 2

A. *Demographic data*
S. T.; 68; female; widowed 2 years; lives in small apartment in city; seen every 6 months by resident at family practice clinic.
B. *Health-illness data*
Health: "not being sick"; illness: "when the bottom falls out of everything." "I'm just not very good anymore; ever since my husband died I haven't been very good. I didn't know how much I depended on him, even when he was sick—my, I sure depended on him. My health just hasn't been as good since he died. I don't sleep as well, and I've lost 20 pounds since my husband died. I spend my time remembering." Says she is not as healthy as most of her friends, but more healthy than those that had to go to nursing homes.

1. Health practices: sleeps four hours, up to bathroom, takes an hour to get back to sleep (listens to radio), sleeps about three more hours; occasionally takes nap after soap opera in afternoon. Not very active; sometimes on nice days walks around block, walks downtown (four blocks one way) about once a week and "looks around"; sometimes gets lunch at the drugstore. Nutrition: "I usually have good breakfasts, but I don't get enough meat. I eat good the days I go to the Senior Center. Other days I just have a cold lunch." 24-hour recall of food intake shows inadequate intake of vegetables. Takes "nerve pills" sometimes at bedtime, sometimes "when I think too much." Is afraid the doctor won't continue to prescribe them. Takes all immunizations when they are offered. Doesn't drink or smoke.
2. Specific health problems: She has no known allergies, says skin much more wrinkled recently. "When my husband was alive he said he didn't care, he loved me the way I was. Now I look at my face, my hands, my arms, my body and think how much more I've aged since he died." Senses "work well"—"my nose works too well, I can't stand it when my neighbor cooks cabbage, and

he cooks cabbage at least once a week." Had to get dentures at age 45—had "soft teeth"; no problems eating whatever she desires. About three years ago started not having a bowel movement every day—"that worries me" takes prune juice sometimes and Milk of Magnesia twice a week—"of course, I feel all washed out the next day after I've used it, but I think I should have a bowel movement every day." Never had any heart or lung problems. Stopped doing breast self-examination two years ago—"I figure if I get sick, it's my time to go." No musculoskeletal problems. Has occasional dizziness and weakness. "Couldn't hold my water" about six years ago, embarrassed, doctor slow to act, husband "told doctor where to go"; surgery corrected problem, "that's one good thing."

C. *Psychological health data*

1. Ego differentiation: not really enjoying life now—"oh, there are some good things, I like my soap opera—I have to follow that family and see what all is happening." Likes a good novel "now and then"—"helps me forget my own troubles when I think about the plot." Likes when grandchildren visit—"but they don't come much anymore, my two daughters live pretty far away; they're busy with their lives, and the kids are in school, so they don't take much time to come and see me, but I understand, they have their lives to live." Life: not better or worse—"the good and the bad balance each other." Glad when husband retired, they traveled one year. "Then he got sick and two years ago he died. Having him sick was better than not having him at all." Sews once a month with group at church, cleans house, crochets sometimes. Says "I guess that's being creative."

2. Body transcendence: changes of body with aging "didn't matter much when my husband was around to tell me he loved me anyway." Doesn't matter much now. "I don't have anybody to care about my body." Doesn't think a change in activity would make her feel different about herself.

3. Ego transcendence: was a good mother and wife; got to go to many of the places she wanted to; liked cooking and raising the children; wishes she had had more so at least one of them would be closer to her. "The things I've accomplished are OK." Sees "some lesson" in loss of husband. "I never thought about goals much, I lived every day as it came, and I guess that's how I'll keep on, and when it's my time to go, I'll go." Thinks maybe if

grandchildren and children were closer, she'd have more of a role in relationship to younger people.

4. Own description of personality: "I'm not sure I have much personality"; good person, did what she was expected to do; had good times in the past.

D. *Economic resource data*

1. Income: Social security—enough to pay the rent, get clothes (sometimes at thrift shop), and "I manage on groceries." Very little for "extras"—"my kids send me money and bring me special gifts of home canned food sometimes."

2. Housing: apartment adequate, secure, comfortable and private ("except for the odors I have to smell"); close to town; grocery store two blocks away.

3. Neighborhood: good, secure, my neighbors check on me, good place for older people.

E. *Cultural and Social Data*

She is respected by people that know her—"hardly anybody comes to me for advice—that might be because my children don't live here." Daughters sometimes ask advice when they call ("they give me advice too"). Instrumental assistance: neighbor who cooks cabbage and two young men from church help with carrying heavy things and washing windows. Affective support: "my husband was my closest friend, but I have another good friend who I see at least twice a month." Talks with daughters at least once a month on the phone, writes letters to daughters once or twice monthly. Sees friends at church about three times a month. No one she sees everyday, but believes neighbors are aware of whether or not she is OK. Groups: church and Senior Center meals.

F. *Physical Examination*

Physical examination reveals a woman who walks slowly with a downcast appearance. She is mildly underweight; vision is good; gross auditory acuity was acceptable, however, she had some wax in her ears, which interfered with the nurse's visualization of the tympanic membranes. Nose was in good condition. Mouth was in good condition, dentures were well cared for but fit loosely. Head and neck: features are symmetrical, she has freedom of movement, there are no lesions or node enlargement, pulses good, and thyroid normal. Breasts revealed no masses. Findings on respiration, circulation, and abdomen were within normal limits. Has kyphosis, but no other musculoskeletal problems. She nearly lost her balance when tested, but the rest of the neurological examination was within normal limits.

G. *Nursing diagnosis*
Coping deficit

· Depression

Impact on Life-style	*Major stressor*
· Few activities, mostly alone	· Unresolved grief; grieving process not completed two years after loss
· Resigned to inevitable death even though she has minimal physical problems	
· Fantasizes about husband's attributes	
Spends a lot of time alone—remembering and "thinking too much"	
· No goals for future activities	
· Little joy in living	
· Perceives health status as "not very good"	

Coping deficit

· Drug dependency

Impact on life-style	*Major stressor*
· Needs to "calm nerves"	· Depression
· Needs help to sleep	
· Believes that daily bowel movement is essential	

Potential coping deficit

· Malnourished

Impact on life-style	*Major stressor*
· Weight loss of 20 lb in two years	· (A more complete nutritional assessment is needed to determine)

Potential coping deficit

· Loneliness

Impact on Life-style	*Major stressor*
· Limited communication with family	· Depression
	Grief
· No regular daily interaction with another person	
· Social network size small—about 12 to 15 people with almost no intimate relationship	

H. *Action*

1. Explore coping deficits with client to seek mutually determined objectives and actions.
2. Refer to social worker, mental health clinic, or public health nurse for follow-up for depression and counselling to deal with grief and preoccupation with loss.
3. Either do a more detailed nutritional assessment or refer to public health nurse or nutritionist for this.
4. Plan a follow-up visit with Mrs. S.T. in four weeks to see if her situation has improved.

The above actions would vary some depending on the nature of the relationship of Mrs. S. T. with the person doing the assessment. If it is an ongoing relationship that includes the intervention component of the nursing process, then the person doing the assessment can carry out some of the actions that might otherwise be referred to the public health nurse.

Mrs. S.T. has some challenges (coping deficits), however, she has the potential skills to facilitate some intervention. Motivation seems very low and her depression is nearly overwhelming her. Although it is not known from the information available, she may be a person who is primarily external in locus of control terms. If so, the loss of her husband and lack of other intimate persons only compounds her needs.

SUMMARY

The foregoing examples are intended to demonstrate how holistic assessment can be done with individual clients. Both Mr. J. G. and Mrs. S. T. can be placed on the health-illness continuum to conceptualize their present health status (see Fig. 11). Although some terminology agreement is recommended in nursing diagnosis, the approach used here is not the only approach that might be effective. It is important to keep in mind when making a diagnosis that data that support it should

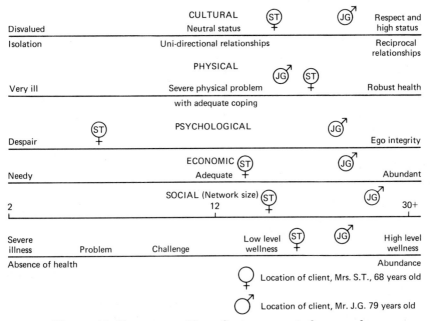

Figure 11. Resource continua for two case study examples.

be as objective as possible (free from the nurse's personal biases), and that cues that a problem exists often come from several categories of the assessment outline when a diagnosis needs to be made.

Holistic assessment is not an easy task. Data collection can sometimes be hampered by environmental distractions or a lack of privacy. The client may provide rather general, nonspecific responses to the nurse's questions. This can be due to a mind-set about history taking based on previous experiences when a client was urged to hurry. Or, the clients may not consider things to which they have adjusted to be significant enough to "bother" the nurse.

Moreover, when a nursing diagnosis is made, a decision about whether something is significant as a problem or whether it is a client uniqueness is often difficult. Maintaining objectivity with the large amount of data required to view the whole person as more than the sum of his or her parts is a continuous challenge for the nurse working with older people.

REFERENCES

1. Sundeen SJ, Stuart G, Rankin ED, et al: *Nurse-Client Interaction: Implementing the Nursing Process.* St. Louis, CV Mosby Company, 1976.

2. Little DE, Carnevali DL: *Nursing Care Planning.* Philadelphia, JB Lippincott Company, 1976, p.156
3. Burgess AW and contributors: *Nursing: Levels of Health Intervention.* Englewood Cliffs, N.J.: Prentice-Hall, 1978.
4. *Standards of Nursing Practice.* Kansas City, Mo, American Nurses' Association, 1973.
5. Pfeiffer E: *Older Americans Resources and Services Multidimensional Functional Assessment Questionnaire.* Durham, NC, Duke University Center for the Study of Aging and Human Development, 1975.
6. Malasanos, Barkauskas, Moss et al: *Health Assessment.* St. Louis, CV Mosby Company, 1977.
7. Bates B: *A Guide to Physical Examination.* Philadelphia, JB Lippincott Company, 1974.

ANNOTATED BIBLIOGRAPHY

Burnside IM (Ed): *Nursing and The Aged.* New York, McGraw-Hill Book Company, 1976.
 A geriatric nursing text that uses normal aging as a baseline to focus on the use of the nursing process with various illnesses and disorders. Physical, mental, and social problems of the aged are covered.
Little DE, Carnevali DL: *Nursing Care Planning,* ed 2. Philadelphia, JB Lippincott Company, 1976.
 An excellent guide to the use of the nursing process. Examples are used to show practical application of theory.
Malasanos, Barkauskas, Moss, et al: *Health Assessment.* St. Louis, CV Mosby Company, 1977.
 A fairly detailed basic text for people learning health history and physical examination skills. This volume focuses on the healthy client and contains many illustrations that effectively demonstrate assessment techniques.
Pfeiffer E: *Multidimensional Functional Assessment: The OARS Methodology–A Manual.* Durham, NC, Duke University Center for the Study of Aging and Human Development. 1975.
 A helpful guide to the use of a rather complete tool to assess the social, economic, mental, and physical health of older people.
Sundeen, SJ, Stuart G, Rankin ED, et al: *Nurse-Client Interaction: Implementing the Nursing Process.* St. Louis, CV Mosby Company, 1976.
 This text presents concepts essential to a holistic approach to nursing practice and contains information on the nurse's self-growth as well as on the essential components of a helping relationship while using the nursing process.

index

Governmental resources, 115
Grandparent, 143
Great Depression, 117
Grieving process, 139

Health, definitions, 58
Health behaviors, 57-58
Health/Illness continuum, 148. *See also*
  Continuum
Health practices, 58
Health problems, 99
Health status, 58, 150
Hearing loss, 73-74
Heart murmurs, 77
Helplessness, 103-104
Heterogeneity, 7-9, 45, 108-109, 139
Hierarchy of needs, 83, 92-93, 94, 102-103.
  See also Needs
Hindu, 53
Hippocrates (460-377 B.C.), 53
History, aging, 3
  American, 132
  medical, 144, 156-157
Holism, 2, 10
Holistic approach, 66
Holistic assessment, *see* Assessment
Holistic perspective, 94
Holistic standpoint, 94
Holistic view, aging, 1-17
  client's, 83
Horticultural/Agricultural societies,
  35-36
Housing, 125
  apartments, 126
  condominiums, 126
  public housing, 118, 119
  retirement houses, 126-127
  retirement villages, 126
Humanism, 11
Humanistic psychology, 102
Human relationships, 96, 100, 135, 151
  intimate, 137, 140
  meaningful, 134
  primary, 133
  secondary, 133
Hunting and gathering societies, 33-35
Hydration, 70

Igbo, of Nigeria, activity orientation,
  27-28
  interdependence, 29
  political system, 38-39

relational orientation, 29
  spiritual ancestors, 31
Immunity, 54
Income maintenance, 121
Independence of elderly, 13, 115, 141
Industrial societies, 36-37, 116
Inspection of skin, 71, 72
Intensity categories, effective, 134-135
  intimate, 134-135
  nominal, 134-135
Interdependence, 133
  Igbo, 29
Intervention, 15
Intervention phase, 62
Isometric exercise, 64, 78

Jews, 32
Judeo-Christian tradition, 32

Keratosis, actinic, 70-71
  seborrheic, 70
Kidneys, 82
Kinship systems, 37-38, 115
Kyphoscoliosis, 79

Label, 7, 8, 13, 15
Legislation (1937), 128
Lentigines, 70
Lewin, Kurt, 133
Life expectancy, 5
Life roles, 143
Life satisfaction, 90, 91
Life span, 5
Life-styles, 8
  transcendent, 110
Locus of control, 103-104, 150
Loneliness, 141, 144
Losses, 3, 12, 53, 111, 135, 139, 151
Loss of taste, 75
Lung capacity, 76

Mabuti pygmies, 34
Masai, 21
Maslow, Abraham, 83, 92-93, 94, 102-103
Medicaid, 118, 124-125, 128
Medical history, 144, 156-157
Medicare, 124-125, 128
Memory, long-range, 80
  loss, 110
  mild, 81
  recent, 80
  transference, 81, 110